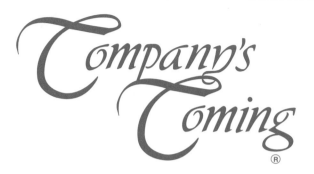

Adding Vegetables
to Everyday Meals

Jean Paré

www.companyscoming.com
visit our website

Front Cover

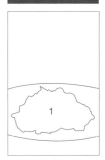

1. Spinach Pesto
   Primavera, page 116

Back Cover

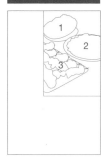

1. Stuffed Tuscan Squash,
   page 67
2. Thai Green Curry Beef,
   page 68
3. Steak and Radish
   Skewers, page 69

First Printing September 2012

Library and Archives Canada Cataloguing in Publication
Paré, Jean, date
Adding vegetables to everyday meals / Jean Paré.
(Original series)
Includes index.
At head of title: Company's Coming.
ISBN 978-1-927126-27-1
1. Cooking (Vegetables). 2. Cookbooks. I. Title.
II. Series: Paré, Jean, date. Original series.
TX801.P36 2012   641.6'5   C2012-900476-6

We gratefully acknowledge the following suppliers for their generous support of our Test and Photography Kitchens:

Broil King Barbecues
Corelle®
Hamilton Beach® Canada
Lagostina®
Proctor Silex® Canada
Tupperware®

Published by
Company's Coming Publishing Limited
2311 – 96 Street
Edmonton, Alberta, Canada T6N 1G3
Tel: 780-450-6223   Fax: 780-450-1857
www.companyscoming.com

Company's Coming is a registered trademark owned by Company's Coming Publishing Limited

We acknowledge the financial support of the Government of Canada through the Canada Book Fund for our publishing activities.

Printed in China

Get more great recipes...FREE!

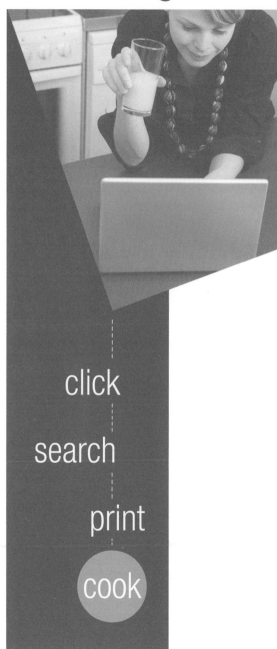
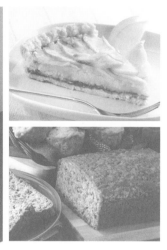

click

search

print

cook

From apple pie to zucchini bread, we've got you covered. Browse our free online recipes for Guaranteed Great!™ results.

You can also sign up to receive our **FREE online newsletter**. You'll receive exclusive offers, FREE recipes and cooking tips, new title previews, and much more...all delivered to your in-box.

So don't delay, visit our website today!

www.companyscoming.com
visit our ⚑ website

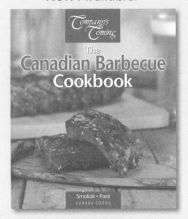
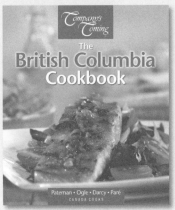
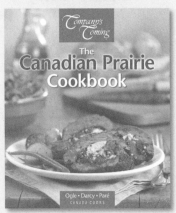
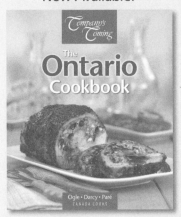
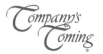

Table of Contents

The Company's Coming Story

Jean Paré (pronounced "jeen PAIR-ee") grew up understanding that the combination of family, friends and home cooking is the best recipe for a good life. From her mother, she learned to appreciate good cooking, while her father praised even her earliest attempts in the kitchen. When Jean left home, she took with her a love of cooking, many family recipes and an intriguing desire to read cookbooks as if they were novels!

"Never share a recipe you wouldn't use yourself."

When her four children had all reached school age, Jean volunteered to cater the 50th anniversary celebration of the Vermilion School of Agriculture, now Lakeland College, in Alberta, Canada. Working out of her home, Jean prepared a dinner for more than 1,000 people, launching a flourishing catering operation that continued for over 18 years. During that time, she had countless opportunities to test new ideas with immediate feedback—resulting in empty plates and contented customers! Whether preparing cocktail sandwiches for a house party or serving a hot meal for 1,500 people, Jean Paré earned a reputation for great food, courteous service and reasonable prices.

As requests for her recipes increased, Jean was often asked the question, "Why don't you write a cookbook?" Jean responded by teaming up with her son, Grant Lovig, in the fall of 1980 to form Company's Coming Publishing Limited. The publication of *150 Delicious Squares* on April 14, 1981 marked the debut of what would soon become one of the world's most popular cookbook series.

The company has grown since those early days when Jean worked from a spare bedroom in her home. Nowadays every Company's Coming recipe is *kitchen-tested* before it is approved for publication.

Company's Coming cookbooks are distributed in Canada, the United States, Australia and other world markets. Bestsellers many times over in English, Company's Coming cookbooks have also been published in French and Spanish.

Familiar and trusted in home kitchens around the world, Company's Coming cookbooks are offered in a variety of formats. Highly regarded as kitchen workbooks, the softcover Original Series, with its lay-flat plastic comb binding, is still a favourite among readers.

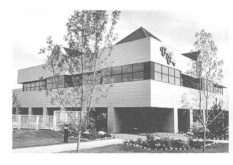

Jean Paré's approach to cooking has always called for *quick and easy recipes* using *everyday ingredients*. That view has served her well. The recipient of many awards, including the Queen Elizabeth Golden Jubilee Medal, Jean was appointed Member of the Order of Canada, her country's highest lifetime achievement honour.

Jean continues to share what she calls The Golden Rule of Cooking: *Never share a recipe you wouldn't use yourself.* It's an approach that has worked—*millions of times over!*

Foreword

You know that you and your family should be getting more vegetables every day, but how do you actually make that happen? *Adding Vegetables* features exactly what the title suggests—easy ways to add vegetables to every single meal of the day, from brunch all the way through to your after-dinner dessert. There's way more than just vegetable side dishes and vegetarian fare here, although those are certainly included!

You'll find a wide range of vegetables in this book, from the standard peas and carrots to more unusual varieties such as bok choy, fennel and kohlrabi. We've also included a few "vegetables" that are technically fruits but that we commonly treat as veggies— think tomatoes and avocadoes.

All of these recipes include healthful veggies. We've used this icon to highlight recipes that include one or more servings of vegetables per portion. You can see page 8 for information about how *Canada's Food Guide* defines a serving of vegetables.

How do you work more vegetables into your daily diet? Well, start your day with Brunch Burritos, then grab a Fennel Beef Bagel for lunch. Down a Super Bunny Smoothie for an afternoon snack that sneaks some carrots into a yummy fruit mix. Below-ground Stew is a comforting and family-friendly dinner option that would go great with a leafy side like Rainbow Spinach Salad. Even dessert can feature vegetables, such as the homey Jicama Pear Crisp or the trendy Spiced Eggplant Cupcakes. Plus you'll find veggie-packed recipes for appetizers, breads, chicken, fish and seafood and much more! Many recipes have been specially designed to be kid-friendly, so you're sure to find something the whole family can enjoy.

Many people grow their own vegetables these days, and fresh veggies are a fantastic option and have a taste that can't be beat! Consider growing them yourself, or check out a farmers' market or your local grocery store's produce section. But don't forget that frozen and canned vegetables count too, and can be a convenient way to work more veggies into your daily life. Often they are as nutritious as fresh vegetables. Frozen vegetables are usually frozen almost immediately after harvest, preserving maximum nutrition.

Start *Adding Vegetables* to your diet today as part of a healthy lifestyle. You'll be glad that you did!

Nutrition Information Guidelines

Each recipe is analyzed using the most current versions of the Canadian Nutrient File from Health Canada, and the United States Department of Agriculture (USDA) Nutrient Database for Standard Reference.

- If more than one ingredient is listed (such as "butter or hard margarine"), or if a range is given (1 – 2 tsp., 5 – 10 mL), only the first ingredient or first amount is analyzed.
- For meat, poultry and fish, the recommended serving size per person is 4 oz. (113 g) uncooked weight (without bone), which is 2 – 3 oz. (57 – 85 g) cooked weight (without bone)—approximately the size of a deck of playing cards.
- Milk used is 1% M.F. (milk fat), unless otherwise stated.
- Cooking oil used is canola oil, unless otherwise stated.
- Ingredients indicating "sprinkle," "optional" or "for garnish" are not included in the nutrition information.
- The fat in recipes and combination foods can vary greatly depending upon the sources and types of fats used in each specific ingredient. For these reasons, the amount of saturated, monounsaturated and polyunsaturated fats may not add up to the total fat content.

Eat Your Veggies

Everyone knows that vegetables are good for you. From the time that we're very small, we're told that spinach will make us strong, that carrots will improve our eyesight and to eat that broccoli "because I told you so!"

Vegetables may not instantly make us as strong as Popeye or give us 20/20 vision, but the more that we learn about nutrition, the more obvious it becomes that vegetables are an essential part of a healthy lifestyle and diet. Vegetables are high in nutrients and vitamins, are more readily available to us today than ever, and even have been shown to prevent and fight disease.

One thing's for certain: it's smart to eat your vegetables.

Canada's Food Guide

Eating Well with Canada's Food Guide recommends that we eat 7 to 10 servings of fruits and vegetables a day. What counts as a vegetable serving?

- ½ cup (125 mL) of fresh, frozen or canned vegetables (such as tomatoes, beans or corn)
- ½ cup (125 mL) cooked leafy vegetables (such as kale)
- 1 cup (250 mL) raw leafy vegetables (such as romaine lettuce)
- ½ cup (125 mL) 100% juice
- 1 fresh, frozen or canned fruit (or ½ cup, 125 mL)

It might initially sound daunting to include 7 to 10 vegetable or fruit servings in your daily diet, but once you start to incorporate them into all your meals throughout the day, you discover it's really not that difficult.

The Vegetable Advantage

The *Food Guide* also suggests eating at least one dark green and one orange vegetable a day. Why do dark green and orange vegetables get preferential treatment? Because they are especially rich in vitamins and nutrients. Dark green veggies (such as asparagus, Brussels sprouts and spinach) are great sources of folate, an important nutrient that has a host of benefits, including a role in cardiovascular health. Bright orange vegetables (such as carrots and squash) are high in beta-carotene, a nutrient that our bodies use to produce vitamin A.

Cruciferous vegetables, which include broccoli, cauliflower, radishes and turnip, are linked with a lower risk of cancer. (The word *cruciferous* comes from Latin and refers to the x-shaped blossoms of these vegetables.) Antioxidants, which are plentiful in vegetables, have been connected with a lower risk of heart disease, cancer and other diseases.

Bland No More

Some methods of preparing vegetables are healthier (and

tastier!) than others. The *Food Guide* favours cooking methods where little to no fat, sugar or salt is added—so, try steaming or grilling those vegetables instead of deep-frying them. Some other healthy alternatives are to sauté, roast or broil your veggies—or even eat them raw as a snack. (Make sure to wash raw vegetables well.)

There's no need to serve bland, uninteresting vegetable dishes. The cooking method that you use can really make vegetables shine. For example, root vegetables (such as sweet potatoes) caramelize when they're cooked, giving them a great, delicately sweet flavour. New potatoes taste fantastic steamed. Bell peppers and asparagus are amazing when they're grilled, and can be perfectly incorporated as a side or as part of the main dish for an early summer barbecue. And instead of adding fatty sauces, consider using fresh herbs and spices to really enhance the flavour of your vegetables.

Eat with the Seasons

Even though these days you can get nearly any food at nearly any time of the year, more and more people are striving to eat more locally grown food and produce. This local-foods movement emphasizes the importance of eating with the seasons—not only does your food not have to be shipped across the country or world, but you're supporting local producers *and*

getting to savour foods at the peak of their freshness at the same time.

Vegetables almost always taste best when they're fresh and in season. Seasonal availability of vegetables depends, of course, on your region and the weather, but here are some general guidelines for when you might expect to find local vegetables:

- Spring: asparagus, fennel, radishes, spinach
- Summer: corn, cucumbers, lettuce, peas, tomatoes
- Fall: carrots, celery, pumpkin, zucchini
- Winter: beets, cabbage, onions

Of course, you can always grow your own vegetables. Whether you have a plot in a community garden, live on a big country farm or have a container of tomatoes on your city balcony, there is no better way to enjoy and appreciate vegetables than to grow your own. Try growing heirloom varieties; most heirloom vegetables are currently not used in large-scale agriculture, usually because they don't store or transport well. But they are often some of the most delicious varieties you'll ever find! Growing heirloom plants in home gardens has become increasingly popular in Europe and North America over the last decade. So consider growing your own.

Curried Pepper Boats

Set your sails for healthier eating—and this is just the recipe to help you do it.
Brightly coloured peppers are packed with flavourful ingredients. Three pepper
boats provide a full serving of vegetables.

Can of chickpeas (garbanzo beans), rinsed and drained	19 oz.	540 mL
Chopped arugula, lightly packed	1 cup	250 mL
Mayonnaise	1/4 cup	60 mL
Cooking oil	1 tbsp.	15 mL
Grated onion	1 tbsp.	15 mL
Finely grated ginger root (or 1/2 tsp., 2 mL, ground ginger)	2 tsp.	10 mL
Lemon juice	1 tsp.	5 mL
Mild curry paste	1 tsp.	5 mL
Brown sugar, packed	1/2 tsp.	2 mL
Chili paste (sambal oelek)	1/2 tsp.	2 mL
Garlic clove, minced (or 1/4 tsp., 1 mL, powder)	1	1
Salt	1/4 tsp.	1 mL
Large yellow peppers, cut into 8 strips each	4	4
Dried cranberries	1/4 cup	60 mL

Process first 12 ingredients in food processor until smooth. Transfer to small bowl.

Spread about 1 tbsp. (15 mL) onto each pepper strip.

Arrange cranberries over top. Makes 32 pepper boats.

1 pepper boat: 35 Calories; 2 g Total Fat (0 g Mono, 0 g Poly, 0 g Sat); 0 mg Cholesterol;
4 g Carbohydrate; trace Fibre; trace Protein; 60 mg Sodium

 HELPFUL HINTS Known by many names, arugula is slightly bitter with a peppery mustard flavour. You may find it in your grocery store sold as Italian cress, rocket, roquette, rugula or rucola.

Savoury Cheesecake with Radish Salsa

Love cheesecake but can't quite wrap your head around a savoury version? It's time to give this trendy food a try. Serve with tortilla chips to complete the experience.

Yellow cornmeal	1/2 cup	125 mL
Butter (or hard margarine), melted	2 tbsp.	30 mL
Large eggs	3	3
Can of white kidney beans, rinsed and drained	19 oz.	540 mL
Cream cheese, softened	8 oz.	250 g
Frozen peas, thawed	1 cup	250 mL
Chili paste (sambal oelek)	2 tsp.	10 mL
Garlic clove, chopped (or 1/4 tsp., 1 mL, powder)	1	1
Salt	1/4 tsp.	1 mL
Pepper	1/4 tsp.	1 mL
Chopped radish	1 cup	250 mL
Chopped ripe (or frozen, thawed) mango	3/4 cup	175 mL
Chopped seeded tomato	3/4 cup	175 mL
Finely chopped red onion	1/4 cup	60 mL
Chopped fresh parsley	2 tbsp.	30 mL
Lemon juice	1 tbsp.	15 mL
Cooking oil	2 tsp.	10 mL
Salt	1/4 tsp.	1 mL
Pepper	1/4 tsp.	1 mL

Combine cornmeal and butter in small bowl. Press firmly in bottom of greased 9 inch (23 cm) deep dish pie plate. Chill for 30 minutes.

Process next 8 ingredients in food processor until smooth. Spread evenly over cornmeal mixture. Bake in 350°F (175°C) oven for about 40 minutes until knife inserted in centre of cheesecake comes out clean. Let stand in pan on wire rack until cool. Chill, covered, for at least 6 hours or overnight.

Combine remaining 9 ingredients in medium bowl. Spoon over cheesecake. Cuts into 12 wedges.

1 wedge: 180 Calories; 11 g Total Fat (1.5 g Mono, 0.5 g Poly, 6 g Sat); 60 mg Cholesterol; 16 g Carbohydrate; 3 g Fibre; 6 g Protein; 330 mg Sodium

Rainbow Cheese Spread

Sneak some extra veggies into your diet with this colourful spread—perfect for serving with crackers.

Cream cheese, softened	8 oz.	250 g
Chopped fresh basil (or 3/4 tsp., 4 mL, dried)	1 tbsp.	15 mL
Goat (chèvre) cheese, cut up	2 oz.	57 g
White wine vinegar	2 tsp.	10 mL
Finely chopped broccoli	1/4 cup	60 mL
Finely chopped carrot	1/4 cup	60 mL
Finely chopped red pepper	1/4 cup	60 mL

Combine first 4 ingredients in medium bowl until smooth.

Add remaining 3 ingredients. Mix well. Chill, covered, for 1 hour. Makes about 2 cups (500 mL).

2 tbsp. (30 mL): 60 Calories; 6 g Total Fat (0 g Mono, 0 g Poly, 3.5 g Sat); 15 mg Cholesterol; trace Carbohydrate; 0 g Fibre; 2 g Protein; 60 mg Sodium

Roasted Red Pepper Hummus

There's no doubt that hummus is popular, but now it's even better with the addition of red pepper for some extra veggie goodness. Serve as a dip with pita bread and vegetables.

Can of white kidney beans, rinsed and drained	19 oz.	540 mL
Jar of roasted red peppers, drained and coarsely chopped	12 oz.	340 mL
Mayonnaise	3 tbsp.	45 mL
Lemon juice	1 tbsp.	15 mL
Garlic clove, chopped (or 1/4 tsp., 1 mL, powder)	1	1
Salt	1/4 tsp.	1 mL
Pepper	1/4 tsp.	1 mL

(continued on next page)

Process all 7 ingredients in food processor until smooth. Makes about 2 1/2 cups (625 mL).

1/4 cup (60 mL): 80 Calories; 3.5 g Total Fat (0 g Mono, 0 g Poly, 0 g Sat); 0 mg Cholesterol; 10 g Carbohydrate; 3 g Fibre; 3 g Protein; 320 mg Sodium

 servings per portion

Baba Ganoush

Roasted garlic provides this spread with a rich yet mellow flavour. Serve chilled or at room temperature with your favourite dippers.

Medium eggplants (about 1 1/4 lbs., 560 g, each)	2	2
Garlic bulb	1	1
Cooking oil	1 tsp.	5 mL
Lemon juice	2 tbsp.	30 mL
Roasted sesame seeds	2 tbsp.	30 mL
Chopped fresh parsley	1 tbsp.	15 mL
Cooking oil	1 tbsp.	15 mL
Salt	3/4 tsp.	4 mL

Chopped fresh parsley, for garnish
Roasted sesame seeds, for garnish

Prick eggplants in several places with a fork. Place on ungreased baking sheet with sides.

Trim 1/4 inch (6 mm) from garlic bulb to expose tops of cloves, leaving bulb intact. Drizzle with first amount of cooking oil. Wrap loosely in foil. Place on same baking sheet. Bake in 425°F (220°C) oven for about 45 minutes until garlic is tender. Remove garlic bulb. Bake eggplants for another 15 minutes until very soft and skins are browned. Let stand for 15 minutes. Cut eggplants in half. Scoop out pulp into food processor. Discard skins. Squeeze garlic bulb to remove cloves from skin. Add to food processor. Discard skin.

Add next 5 ingredients. Process until smooth. Transfer to serving bowl. Cool.

Garnish with parsley and sesame seeds. Makes about 2 cups (500 mL).

1/4 cup (60 mL): 80 Calories; 3.5 g Total Fat (2 g Mono, 1 g Poly, 0 g Sat); 0 mg Cholesterol; 11 g Carbohydrate; 5 g Fibre; 2 g Protein; 240 mg Sodium

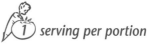

Spinach Edamame Dip

Protein-packed edamame makes the perfect partner for spinach in this vibrant dip. Serve with toasted pita chips, wheat crackers or vegetable sticks.

Water	3 cups	750 mL
Frozen shelled edamame (soybeans)	2 cups	500 mL
Chopped fresh spinach leaves, lightly packed	1 cup	250 mL
Sour cream	1/3 cup	75 mL
Roasted sesame seeds	2 tbsp.	30 mL
Lemon juice	1 tbsp.	15 mL
Garlic clove, chopped (or 1/4 tsp., 1 mL, powder)	1	1
Salt	1/2 tsp.	2 mL
Pepper	1/4 tsp.	1 mL
Roasted sesame seeds	2 tsp.	10 mL

Bring water to a boil in medium saucepan. Add edamame. Reduce heat to medium. Boil gently, uncovered, for 5 minutes. Drain, reserving 1/4 cup (60 mL) cooking water. Rinse edamame with cold water. Drain well. Transfer to food processor.

Add next 7 ingredients and reserved cooking water. Process until smooth. Transfer to serving bowl.

Sprinkle with second amount of sesame seeds. Makes about 2 cups (500 mL).

1/4 cup (60 mL): 80 Calories; 4.5 g Total Fat (1 g Mono, 0.5 g Poly, 1.5 g Sat); trace Cholesterol; 5 g Carbohydrate; 2 g Fibre; 4 g Protein; 130 mg Sodium

Pictured on page 17.

 HELPFUL HINTS *Edamame* is the Japanese name for fresh soybeans. Edamame are known for their plump size and nutty flavour, and they're great as a snack on their own or added to recipes.

Shrimp Veggie Salad Rolls

These refreshing and colourful rolls can be made a few hours in advance and chilled until you're ready to serve them. Just arrange them on a plate, spaced a bit apart, and cover them with a damp towel and plastic wrap. Each roll contains half a serving of vegetables.

Lime juice	1 tbsp.	15 mL
Water	1 tbsp.	15 mL
Soy sauce	2 tsp.	10 mL
Granulated sugar	1 tsp.	5 mL
Chili paste (sambal oelek)	1/2 tsp.	2 mL
Salt	1/8 tsp.	0.5 mL
Grated carrot	1 cup	250 mL
Julienned English cucumber (with peel), see Tip, below	1 cup	250 mL
Julienned yellow turnip (rutabaga), see Tip, below	1 cup	250 mL
Chopped fresh cilantro (or parsley)	2 tbsp.	30 mL
Chopped fresh mint	2 tbsp.	30 mL
Rice paper rounds (6 inch, 15 cm, diameter)	12	12
Cooked large shrimp (peeled and deveined), halved lengthwise	18	18

Stir first 6 ingredients in medium bowl until sugar is dissolved.

Add next 5 ingredients. Toss.

Place 1 rice paper round in shallow bowl of hot water until just softened. Place on work surface. Arrange 3 shrimp halves across centre. Top with about 3 tbsp. (45 mL) carrot mixture. Fold sides over filling. Roll up tightly from bottom to enclose. Transfer to serving plate. Cover with damp towel to prevent drying. Repeat with remaining rice paper rounds, shrimp and carrot mixture. Makes 12 rolls.

1 roll: 70 Calories; 0 g Total Fat (0 g Mono, 0 g Poly, 0 g Sat); 40 mg Cholesterol; 11 g Carbohydrate; 0 g Fibre; 5 g Protein; 230 mg Sodium

Pictured on page 17.

 tip   To julienne, cut into very thin strips that resemble matchsticks.

Pepper Roll-ups

These tasty rolls are packed with colourful peppers and cream-cheesy filling with a mild chili heat. You can use any colour of peppers you like depending upon what you've got on hand.

Cream cheese, softened	3/4 cup	175 mL
Pizza sauce	2 tbsp.	30 mL
Dried crushed chilies	1/8 tsp.	0.5 mL
Salt	1/8 tsp.	0.5 mL
Whole-wheat flour tortillas (10 inch, 25 cm, diameter)	4	4
Finely chopped green pepper	2/3 cup	150 mL
Finely chopped orange pepper	2/3 cup	150 mL
Finely chopped red pepper	2/3 cup	150 mL

Combine first 4 ingredients in small bowl.

Spread over tortillas, almost to edge.

Scatter remaining 3 ingredients over top. Roll up tightly, jelly-roll style. Wrap in plastic wrap. Chill for 2 hours. Trim ends. Cut each roll into 10 slices. Makes 40 roll-ups.

1 roll-up: 35 Calories; 1.5 g Total Fat (0 g Mono, 0 g Poly, 1 g Sat); trace Cholesterol; 4 g Carbohydrate; trace Fibre; trace Protein; 70 mg Sodium

Pictured at right.

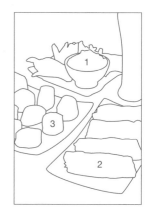

1. Spinach Edamame Dip, page 14
2. Shrimp Veggie Salad Rolls, page 15
3. Pepper Roll-ups, above

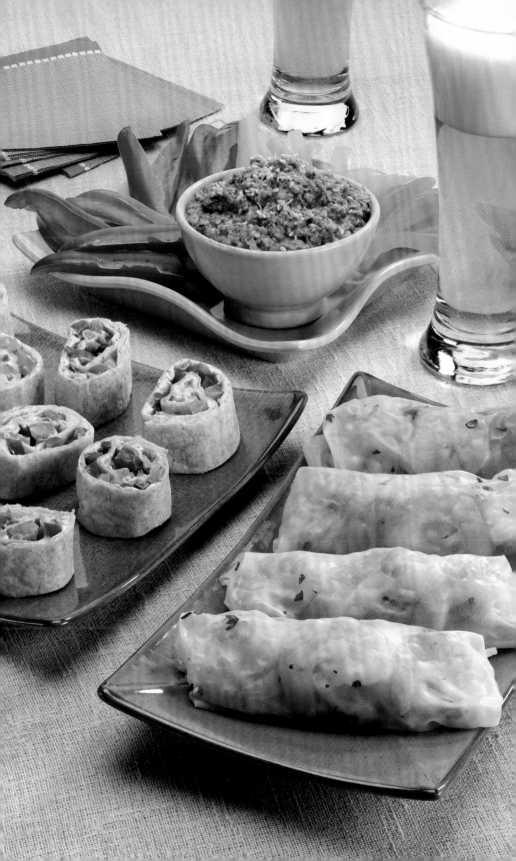

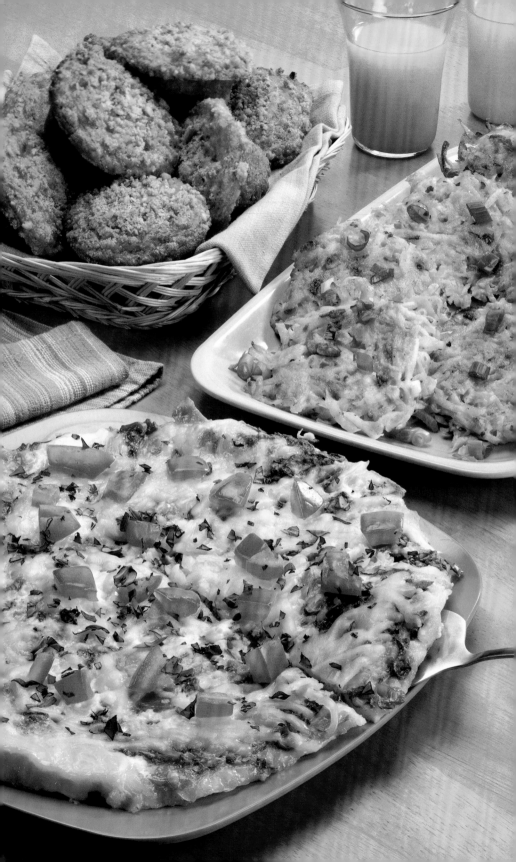

Corn Nachos

*These are not your usual nachos. These are loaded with veggies for a boost
of vitamins and nutrients, taking snacking to a whole new level! And if
you serve them with salsa, you'll add even more vegetables.*

Bag of tortilla chips	11 1/2 oz.	300 g
Can of kernel corn, drained	7 oz.	199 mL
Chopped red pepper	1/2 cup	125 mL
Chopped green onion	1/4 cup	60 mL
Chili powder	1 tsp.	5 mL
Grated Mexican cheese blend	2 cups	500 mL

Arrange half of tortilla chips in ungreased 9 x 13 inch (23 x 33 cm)
baking dish.

Toss next 4 ingredients in medium bowl. Scatter half over tortilla chips.

Sprinkle with half of cheese. Repeat with remaining tortilla chips, corn
mixture and cheese. Bake in 400°F (200°C) oven for about 10 minutes until
cheese is melted. Serves 8.

*1 serving: 320 Calories; 18 g Total Fat (6 g Mono, 1.5 g Poly, 7 g Sat); 25 mg Cholesterol;
32 g Carbohydrate; 3 g Fibre; 9 g Protein; 460 mg Sodium*

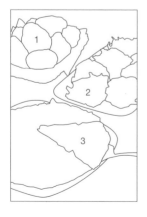

1. Rhubarb Streusel Muffins, page 48
2. Potato Squash Latkes, page 24
3. Green Eggs and Prosciutto, page 25

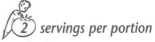

Gazpacho Smoothie

If you enjoy vegetable cocktail drinks, you're going to love this savoury and refreshing smoothie that's loaded with all the flavours of the popular Spanish soup.

Chopped English cucumber (with peel)	2 cups	500 mL
Can of diced tomatoes (with juice)	14 oz.	398 mL
Unsweetened applesauce	1/2 cup	125 mL
Chopped red pepper	1/4 cup	60 mL
Chopped fresh cilantro (or parsley)	1 tbsp.	15 mL
Pepper	1/4 tsp.	1 mL
Garlic powder	1/8 tsp.	0.5 mL
Onion powder	1/8 tsp.	0.5 mL
Hot pepper sauce (optional)	1/8 tsp.	0.5 mL

Process all 9 ingredients in blender until smooth. Makes about 3 1/3 cups (825 mL). Serves 4.

1 serving: 45 Calories; 0 g Total Fat (0 g Mono, 0 g Poly, 0 Sat); 0 mg Cholesterol; 11 g Carbohydrate; 1 g Fibre; 1 g Protein; 310 mg Sodium

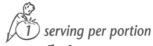 *1 serving per portion*

Super Bunny Smoothie

Get your morning off to a good start with this thick, creamy and not-too-sweet smoothie. You could cook extra carrots at dinnertime so you're all ready to go in the morning.

Chopped carrot	2 cups	500 mL
Ice water		
Frozen overripe medium banana, cut up (see Tip, page 22)	1	1
Whole frozen strawberries	1 cup	250 mL
Milk	3/4 cup	175 mL
Vanilla yogurt	3/4 cup	175 mL
Liquid honey	2 tsp.	10 mL

(continued on next page)

Pour water into small saucepan until about 1 inch (2.5 cm) deep. Add carrot. Cover. Bring to a boil. Reduce heat to medium. Boil gently for about 10 minutes until tender. Drain.

Plunge into ice water in medium bowl. Let stand for about 10 minutes until cold. Drain. Transfer to blender or food processor.

Add remaining 5 ingredients. Process until smooth. Makes about 3 1/2 cups (875 mL). Serves 4.

1 serving: 130 Calories; 2.5 g Total Fat (0 g Mono, 0 g Poly, 1 g Sat); 5 mg Cholesterol; 26 g Carbohydrate; 3 g Fibre; 5 g Protein; 105 mg Sodium

Veggie "Chips" and Guacamole

If chips and dip are your guilty pleasure, this might be just the solution for you. This spicy guacamole is served with sliced veggies for a guilt-free snacking experience.

Mashed avocado	1 1/2 cups	375 mL
Chopped seeded tomato	1/2 cup	125 mL
Finely chopped yellow pepper	1/4 cup	60 mL
Thinly sliced green onion	3 tbsp.	45 mL
Lime juice	2 tbsp.	30 mL
Chopped fresh cilantro (or parsley)	1 tbsp.	15 mL
Cooking oil	2 tsp.	10 mL
Finely diced fresh hot chili pepper (see Tip, page 47)	1/4 tsp.	1 mL
Garlic clove, minced (or 1/4 tsp., 1 mL, powder)	1	1
Salt	1/2 tsp.	2 mL
Pepper	1/4 tsp.	1 mL
Small peeled jicama, quartered and thinly sliced (about 1/8 inch, 3 mm, slices)	1	1
Orange pepper pieces (1 inch, 2.5 cm)	1 cup	250 mL
Diagonally sliced zucchini (with peel), about 1/4 inch (6 mm) slices	1 cup	250 mL

Combine first 11 ingredients in medium bowl.

Serve with remaining 3 ingredients. Serves 12.

1 serving: 60 Calories; 4.5 g Total Fat (3 g Mono, 0.5 g Poly, 0.5 g Sat); 0 mg Cholesterol; 6 g Carbohydrate; 3 g Fibre; trace Protein; 85 mg Sodium

Carrot Cake Cookies

When it comes to veggies, every bit counts. Kids will love these cute little cookies, and you can serve them with confidence knowing that they're getting nutritious fruit and vegetables with every bite.

All-purpose flour	2 cups	500 mL
Quick-cooking rolled oats	1/2 cup	125 mL
Baking soda	1 tsp.	5 mL
Ground cinnamon	1/2 tsp.	2 mL
Ground ginger	1/2 tsp.	2 mL
Salt	1/2 tsp.	2 mL
Butter (or hard margarine), softened	1/2 cup	125 mL
Granulated sugar	3/4 cup	175 mL
Large egg	1	1
Buttermilk (or soured milk, see Tip, page 60)	1/4 cup	60 mL
Vanilla extract	1 tsp.	5 mL
Grated carrot	1 cup	250 mL
Dark raisins	1/2 cup	125 mL

Combine first 6 ingredients in medium bowl.

Beat butter and sugar in large bowl until light and fluffy. Add next 3 ingredients. Beat well. Add flour mixture in 2 additions, mixing well after each addition, until no dry flour remains.

Add carrot and raisins. Mix well. Drop, using 1 tbsp. (15 mL) for each, about 1 inch (2.5 cm) apart, onto greased cookie sheets. Bake in 375°F (190°C) oven for about 10 minutes until puffed and golden on edges. Let stand on cookie sheets for 5 minutes before removing to wire racks to cool. Makes about 38 cookies.

1 cookie: 80 Calories; 2.5 g Total Fat (0.5 g Mono, 0 g Poly, 1.5 g Sat); 10 mg Cholesterol; 12 g Carbohydrate; 0 g Fibre; 1 g Protein; 80 mg Sodium

 tip When your bananas get too ripe to enjoy fresh, peel and cut them into 2 inch (5 cm) chunks and freeze on a baking sheet. Once frozen, transfer to freezer bag for use in any blended beverage. Ripe bananas have superior flavour for beverages.

Pumpkin Pecan Waffles

Warm and welcoming waffles will lure your brunch guests into the kitchen.
Keep your waffles warm in the oven until they're all cooked and ready to serve.

All-purpose flour	1 1/2 cups	375 mL
Finely chopped pecans, toasted	1/2 cup	125 mL
(see Tip, page 38)		
Whole-wheat flour	1/2 cup	125 mL
Brown sugar, packed	2 tbsp.	30 mL
Baking powder	2 tsp.	10 mL
Baking soda	1/2 tsp.	2 mL
Ground cinnamon	1/2 tsp.	2 mL
Ground ginger	1/2 tsp.	2 mL
Salt	1/4 tsp.	1 mL
Large eggs, fork-beaten	2	2
Canned pure pumpkin (no spices),	1 cup	250 mL
(see Tip, below)		
Milk	1 cup	250 mL
Orange juice	1/2 cup	125 mL
Cooking oil	1/4 cup	60 mL
Grated orange zest (see Tip, page 97)	1/2 tsp.	2 mL

Combine first 9 ingredients in large bowl. Make a well in centre.

Combine remaining 6 ingredients in medium bowl. Add to well. Stir until just moistened. Batter will be lumpy. Preheat waffle iron. Spray with cooking spray. Pour batter onto greased waffle iron, using 2/3 to 1 cup (150 to 250 mL) for each waffle. Cook for 3 to 5 minutes per batch until browned and crisp. Transfer to plate. Cover to keep warm. Repeat with remaining batter, spraying waffle iron with cooking spray if necessary to prevent sticking. Makes about 5 Belgian waffles or 8 regular waffles.

1 Belgian waffle: 450 Calories; 22 g Total Fat (12 g Mono, 6 g Poly, 2.5 g Sat); 55 mg Cholesterol; 54 g Carbohydrate; 6 g Fibre; 12 g Protein; 390 mg Sodium

 tip Store any leftover pumpkin in an airtight container in the refrigerator for 3 to 5 days or in the freezer for up to 12 months.

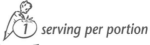

Potato Squash Latkes

Potato latkes with the added goodness of squash and tasty green onion.
Serve with sour cream, plain yogurt or applesauce.

Large egg	1	1
All-purpose flour	1/4 cup	60 mL
Chopped fresh parsley	1 tbsp.	15 mL
(or 3/4 tsp., 4 mL, flakes)		
Salt	1/4 tsp.	1 mL
Pepper	1/4 tsp.	1 mL
Grated peeled baking potato,	2 cups	500 mL
squeezed dry		
Grated butternut squash (see Tip,	1 1/2 cups	375 mL
page 33)		
Thinly sliced green onion	1/4 cup	60 mL
Cooking oil	6 tbsp.	100 mL

Whisk first 5 ingredients in large bowl.

Add next 3 ingredients. Stir.

Heat 2 tbsp. (30 mL) cooking oil in large frying pan on medium. Drop 4 portions of potato mixture into pan, using about 1/4 cup (60 mL) for each. Press down lightly to 3 inch (7.5 cm) diameter. Cook for about 3 minutes per side until browned. Transfer to paper towel–lined plate to drain. Cover to keep warm. Repeat with remaining cooking oil and potato mixture. Makes about 12 latkes. Serves 6.

1 serving: 170 Calories; 11 g Total Fat (7 g Mono, 3 g Poly, 1 g Sat); 25 mg Cholesterol;
17 g Carbohydrate; 2 g Fibre; 3 g Protein; 90 mg Sodium

Pictured on page 18.

Green Eggs and Prosciutto

You've surely heard of this whimsical dish being served with ham, but we're certain it's even better with prosciutto.

Cooking oil	1 tsp.	5 mL
Chopped prosciutto (or deli) ham	3/4 cup	175 mL
Chopped arugula, lightly packed	1 1/2 cups	375 mL
Chopped green onion	2 tbsp.	30 mL
Large eggs	8	8
Salt	1/8 tsp.	0.5 mL
Pepper, just a pinch		
Grated Italian cheese blend	1/2 cup	125 mL
Chopped Roma (plum) tomato	1/4 cup	60 mL
Chopped fresh basil	2 tsp.	10 mL

Heat cooking oil in large non-stick frying pan on medium. Add prosciutto. Cook for 1 minute, stirring occasionally.

Add arugula and green onion. Cook for about 2 minutes, stirring occasionally, until arugula is wilted.

Whisk next 3 ingredients in medium bowl. Pour over arugula mixture. Reduce heat to medium-low. Cook, covered, for about 15 minutes until bottom is golden and top is set. Remove from heat.

Sprinkle with cheese. Let stand, covered, for about 1 minute until cheese is melted.

Scatter tomato and basil over top. Cuts into 6 wedges. Serves 6.

1 serving: 150 Calories; 9 g Total Fat (2.5 g Mono, 1 g Poly, 3 g Sat); 200 mg Cholesterol; 1 g Carbohydrate; 0 g Fibre; 14 g Protein; 680 mg Sodium

Pictured on page 18.

 HELPFUL HINTS Prosciutto is a type of ham that is generally seasoned, salt-cured and dried. The meat is then processed, which gives it a firm, dense texture.

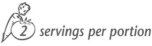

Brunch Burritos

These big, filling burritos are sure to satisfy those with hefty appetites.
Loaded with scrambled egg, avocado and lots of vegetables.

Cooking oil	2 tsp.	10 mL
Sliced onion	1 cup	250 mL
Sliced red pepper	1 cup	250 mL
Sliced yellow pepper	1 cup	250 mL
Sliced zucchini (with peel)	1 cup	250 mL
Chili powder	1 tsp.	5 mL
Ground cumin	1/2 tsp.	2 mL
Garlic clove, minced	1	1
(or 1/4 tsp., 1 mL, powder)		
Salt	1/4 tsp.	1 mL
Pepper	1/4 tsp.	1 mL
Cooking oil	1 tsp.	5 mL
Large eggs	6	6
Milk	1/4 cup	60 mL
Flour tortillas (9 inch, 23 cm, diameter)	4	4
Chopped avocado	1/2 cup	125 mL
Grated jalapeño Monterey Jack cheese	1/3 cup	75 mL
Bacon slices, cooked crisp and crumbled	4	4
Salsa	1/4 cup	60 mL

Heat cooking oil in large frying pan on medium. Add next 9 ingredients. Cook for about 8 minutes, stirring often, until onion is softened. Transfer to medium bowl. Cover to keep warm. Wipe frying pan with paper towel.

Heat second amount of cooking oil in same frying pan on medium. Whisk eggs and milk in small bowl. Add to frying pan. Reduce heat to medium-low. Stir slowly and constantly with spatula while starting to set, scraping sides and bottom of pan until eggs are set and liquid is evaporated.

Arrange egg mixture along centre of each tortilla. Spoon onion mixture over egg.

Top with remaining 4 ingredients. Fold sides over filling. Roll up from bottom to enclose. Makes 4 burritos. Serves 4.

1 serving: *510 Calories; 24 g Total Fat (11 g Mono, 3.5 g Poly, 7 g Sat); 225 mg Cholesterol;*
53 g Carbohydrate; 6 g Fibre; 21 g Protein; 830 mg Sodium

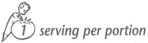 *serving per portion*

Fennel Beef Bagels

Versatile bagels are the perfect base for tasty toppings of cheese, fennel, tomato and deli roast beef. These open-faced sandwiches are a satisfying brunch or lunch option. Great baked or unbaked—try them both ways!

Cooking oil	1 tsp.	5 mL
Thinly sliced fennel bulb (white part only)	3 cups	750 mL
Mayonnaise	3 tbsp.	45 mL
Garlic powder, sprinkle		
Onion bagels, split	2	2
Deli roast beef slices (about 6 oz., 170 g)	4	4
Large tomato slices	4	4
Havarti cheese slices (about 4 oz., 113 g)	4	4

Heat cooking oil in medium frying pan on medium. Add fennel. Cook for about 10 minutes, stirring often, until fennel is softened and starting to brown.

Combine mayonnaise and garlic powder in small bowl. Spread over bagel halves. Arrange cut-side up on ungreased baking sheet.

Layer beef, fennel, tomato and cheese, in order given, over top. Bake in 350°F (175°C) oven for about 10 minutes until cheese is melted and bagel starts to brown on edges. Makes 4 open-faced bagels. Serves 4.

1 serving: 410 Calories; 22 g Total Fat (2.5 g Mono, 0 g Poly, 9 g Sat); 60 mg Cholesterol; 32 g Carbohydrate; 3 g Fibre; 20 g Protein; 910 mg Sodium

HELPFUL HINTS

Fennel, a member of the parsley family, offers a sweet, light licorice flavour that is similar to anise but less intense. The broad bulb and celery-like stems can be enjoyed raw or cooked; however, fennel's aromatic punch is lessened through cooking. When choosing fennel, look for bulbs that have no signs of browning and crisp, unblemished stalks and leaves.

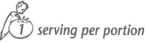

Bruschetta Strata

Stratas take a little advance planning since they need to be assembled the night before, but we can assure you that the fresh bruschetta flavours in this unique offering are well worth the wait.

Cooking oil	1 tsp.	5 mL
Chopped zucchini (with peel)	2 cups	500 mL
Chopped onion	1 cup	250 mL
Garlic cloves, minced	2	2
(or 1/2 tsp., 2 mL, powder)		
Salt, sprinkle		
French bread slices (1/2 inch, 12 mm, each)	12	12
Large eggs	6	6
Milk	1 cup	250 mL
Dried oregano	1 tsp.	5 mL
Salt	1/8 tsp.	0.5 mL
Pepper	1/8 tsp.	0.5 mL
Chopped Roma (plum) tomato	1 cup	250 mL
Grated Parmesan cheese	1/4 cup	60 mL
Chopped fresh basil	2 tbsp.	30 mL

Heat cooking oil in large frying pan on medium. Add next 4 ingredients. Cook for about 8 minutes, stirring often, until vegetables start to brown.

Arrange bread slices, slightly overlapping, in greased 9 x 13 inch (23 x 33 cm) baking dish. Spoon zucchini mixture over bread slices.

Whisk next 5 ingredients in medium bowl. Pour over top. Chill, covered, for at least 6 hours or overnight. Bake, uncovered, in 350°F (175°C) oven for about 40 minutes until puffed and golden.

Scatter remaining 3 ingredients over top. Serves 6.

1 serving: 250 Calories; 7 g Total Fat (3 g Mono, 1 g Poly, 2 g Sat); 140 mg Cholesterol; 35 g Carbohydrate; 3 g Fibre; 13 g Protein; 450 mg Sodium

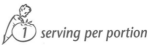

Tomato Corn Cobbler

Turn the whole family into cobbler gobblers when you set this tasty comfort food out for brunch.

Chopped seeded tomato	2 1/2 cups	625 mL
Chopped fresh (or frozen, thawed) kernel corn	1 1/2 cups	375 mL
Finely chopped green onion	2 tbsp.	30 mL
Butter (or hard margarine), melted	1 tbsp.	15 mL
Salt	1/8 tsp.	0.5 mL
Pepper	1/8 tsp.	0.5 mL
Chopped fresh basil (or 3/4 tsp., 4 mL, dried)	1 tbsp.	15 mL
All-purpose flour	1 cup	250 mL
Baking powder	2 tsp.	10 mL
Grated lemon zest	1/2 tsp.	2 mL
Salt	1/4 tsp.	1 mL
Cold butter (or hard margarine), cut up	1/3 cup	75 mL
Large egg, fork-beaten	1	1
Milk	2/3 cup	150 mL
Grated sharp Cheddar cheese	1/2 cup	125 mL

Combine first 6 ingredients in microwave-safe 8 x 8 inch (20 x 20 cm) baking dish. Microwave, covered, on high (100%) for about 4 minutes until heated through (see Tip, page 119).

Add basil. Stir.

Combine next 4 ingredients in medium bowl. Cut in butter until mixture resembles coarse crumbs. Make a well in centre.

Add remaining 3 ingredients to well. Stir until just moistened. Drop by mounded spoonfuls over hot tomato mixture. Bake in 400°F (200°C) oven for about 30 minutes until golden and wooden pick inserted in centre of biscuit comes out clean. Serves 6.

1 serving: 290 Calories; 17 g Total Fat (4.5 g Mono, 1 g Poly, 10 g Sat); 65 mg Cholesterol; 28 g Carbohydrate; 2 g Fibre; 8 g Protein; 390 mg Sodium

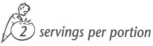

Portobello Pizzas

Are your pizzas boring? Perhaps that's because you're still using dough.
Portobello caps packed with rice and pizza toppings are a new alternative.

Portobello mushrooms (about 4 inch, 10 cm, diameter), stems and gills removed (see Tip, page 136)	4	4
Cooking oil	1 tbsp.	15 mL
Salt	1/4 tsp.	1 mL
Pepper	1/8 tsp.	0.5 mL
Cooking oil	2 tsp.	10 mL
Finely chopped onion	1/2 cup	125 mL
Chopped deli ham	1/4 cup	60 mL
Cooked long-grain white rice	1/2 cup	125 mL
Grated Swiss cheese	1/2 cup	125 mL
Chopped fresh parsley (or 3/4 tsp., 4 mL, flakes)	1 tbsp.	15 mL
Grated Swiss cheese	1/4 cup	60 mL

Brush mushrooms with first amount of cooking oil. Sprinkle with salt and pepper. Place mushrooms, stem-side up, on greased baking sheet.

Heat second amount of cooking oil in large frying pan on medium. Add onion and ham. Cook for about 5 minutes, stirring often, until onion is softened. Remove from heat.

Add next 3 ingredients. Stir well. Spoon into mushroom caps. Cover with greased foil. Bake in 375°F (190°C) oven for 10 minutes. Carefully remove foil.

Sprinkle second amount of cheese over top. Bake for about 10 minutes until mushrooms are tender and cheese is melted. Makes 4 pizzas. Serves 4.

1 serving: 210 Calories; 11 g Total Fat (4.5 g Mono, 2 g Poly, 3.5 g Sat); 20 mg Cholesterol; 20 g Carbohydrate; 4 g Fibre; 12 g Protein; 280 mg Sodium

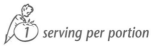

Nutty Salad Rolls

No one will think you're nutty when you serve these delicious salad rolls.
Curried peanut sauce blends perfectly with refreshing salad ingredients, all
packed into soft rice wraps.

Cooking oil	2 tsp.	10 mL
Lean ground beef	1 lb.	454 g
Chopped onion	1/2 cup	125 mL
Mild curry paste	1 tbsp.	15 mL
Smooth peanut butter	1/2 cup	125 mL
Plain yogurt	1/3 cup	75 mL
Lime juice	3 tbsp.	45 mL
Soy sauce	2 tbsp.	30 mL
Chili paste (sambal oelek)	1 tsp.	5 mL
Shredded lettuce, lightly packed	3 cups	750 mL
Chopped fresh bean sprouts	2 cups	500 mL
Grated carrot	1/2 cup	125 mL
Finely shredded basil	1/3 cup	75 mL
Rice paper rounds (9 inch, 23 cm, diameter)	12	12

Heat cooking oil in large frying pan on medium-high. Add beef and onion. Scramble-fry for about 10 minutes until beef is no longer pink.

Add curry paste. Heat and stir for 1 minute. Transfer to large bowl. Cool.

Combine next 5 ingredients in small bowl. Add to beef mixture. Stir.

Add next 4 ingredients. Stir well.

Place 1 rice paper round in shallow bowl of hot water until just softened. Place on work surface. Spoon about 1/3 cup (75 mL) lettuce mixture along centre. Fold sides over filling. Roll up tightly from bottom to enclose. Transfer to serving plate. Cover with damp towel to prevent drying. Repeat with remaining rice paper rounds and lettuce mixture. Makes 12 rolls. Serves 6.

1 serving: 440 Calories; 25 g Total Fat (6 g Mono, 1 g Poly, 7 g Sat); 45 mg Cholesterol;
30 g Carbohydrate; 4 g Fibre; 23 g Protein; 780 mg Sodium

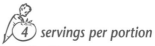

Roasted Tomato Basil Soup

The ideal match—deeply flavoured roasted tomatoes with fresh basil.
This light soup makes the perfect starter for a fancy meal.

Roma (plum) tomatoes, halved and seeds removed	3 lbs.	1.4 kg
Chopped onion	1 cup	250 mL
Cooking oil	1 tbsp.	15 mL
Garlic cloves	3	3
Salt	1/4 tsp.	1 mL
Pepper	1/4 tsp.	1 mL
Prepared chicken broth	2 cups	500 mL
Tomato paste (see Tip, below)	2 tbsp.	30 mL
Brown sugar, packed	4 tsp.	20 mL
Chopped fresh basil	2 tbsp.	30 mL

Toss first 6 ingredients in large bowl until coated. Arrange in single layer on greased baking sheet with sides. Cook in 400°F (200°C) oven for about 40 minutes until tomato starts to brown on edges. Transfer to blender or food processor. Carefully process until smooth (see Safety Tip). Transfer to large saucepan.

Add next 3 ingredients. Stir. Bring to a boil. Reduce heat to medium-low. Simmer, uncovered, for 20 minutes, stirring occasionally, to blend flavours.

Add basil. Stir. Makes about 4 1/4 cups (1 L). Serves 4.

1 serving: 140 Calories; 4 g Total Fat (2.5 g Mono, 1.5 g Poly, 0 g Sat); 0 mg Cholesterol; 25 g Carbohydrate; 5 g Fibre; 4 g Protein; 440 mg Sodium

Pictured on page 35.

Safety Tip: Follow manufacturer's instructions for processing hot liquids.

 tip   If a recipe calls for less than an entire can of tomato paste, freeze the unopened can for 30 minutes. Open both ends and push the contents through one end. Slice off only what you need. Freeze the remaining paste in a resealable freezer bag or plastic wrap for future use.

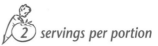

Creamy Butternut Squash Soup

Mild and delicious butternut squash flavour in a creamy fall-inspired soup.
This veggie-rich recipe pairs nicely with whole-grain bread.

Cooking oil	1 tsp.	5 mL
Chopped onion	1 cup	250 mL
Garlic cloves, chopped	2	2
(or 1/2 tsp., 2 mL, powder)		
Chopped butternut squash (see Tip, below)	4 cups	1 L
Prepared chicken broth	3 cups	750 mL
Salt	1/8 tsp.	0.5 mL
Pepper	1/4 tsp.	1 mL
Half-and-half cream	1 cup	250 mL

Heat cooking oil in large saucepan on medium. Add onion and garlic. Cook for about 5 minutes, stirring often, until onion is softened.

Add next 4 ingredients. Stir. Bring to a boil. Reduce heat to medium-low. Simmer, covered, for about 25 minutes until squash is tender. Carefully process with hand blender, or in blender in batches, until smooth (see Safety Tip). Return to same pot.

Add cream. Stir. Makes about 6 1/3 cups (1.6 L). Serves 4.

1 serving: 180 Calories; 8 g Total Fat (2.5 g Mono, 0.5 g Poly, 4.5 g Sat); 20 mg Cholesterol; 26 g Carbohydrate; 3 g Fibre; 4 g Protein; 530 mg Sodium

Pictured on page 35.

Safety Tip: Follow manufacturer's instructions for processing hot liquids.

 Some people have an allergic reaction to raw squash flesh, so wear rubber gloves when cutting or handling raw butternut squash or acorn squash.

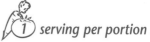

Kohlrabi Pepper Slaw

Fresh, crunchy and sweet—just the traits you're looking for in a successful slaw recipe. Lovely notes of mint and a slight chili heat tie everything together.

Chopped fresh mint	2 tbsp.	30 mL
(or 1 1/2 tsp., 7 mL, dried)		
Cooking oil	1 tbsp.	15 mL
Lime juice	1 tbsp.	15 mL
Liquid honey	1 tbsp.	15 mL
Soy sauce	1 tbsp.	15 mL
Dried crushed chilies	1/8 tsp.	0.5 mL
Garlic powder	1/8 tsp.	0.5 mL
Salt	1/8 tsp.	0.5 mL
Julienned kohlrabi (see Tip, page 15)	2 cups	500 mL
Fresh bean sprouts	1 cup	250 mL
Slivered red pepper	1 cup	250 mL
Grated carrot	1/2 cup	125 mL
Thinly sliced green onion	2 tbsp.	30 mL

Whisk first 8 ingredients in large bowl.

Add remaining 5 ingredients. Stir. Makes about 6 cups (1.5 L). Serves 6.

*1 serving: 50 Calories; 2.5 g Total Fat (1.5 g Mono, 0.5 g Poly, 0 g Sat); 0 mg Cholesterol;
8 g Carbohydrate; 2 g Fibre; 2 g Protein; 210 mg Sodium*

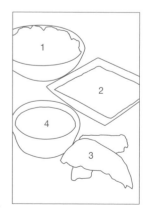

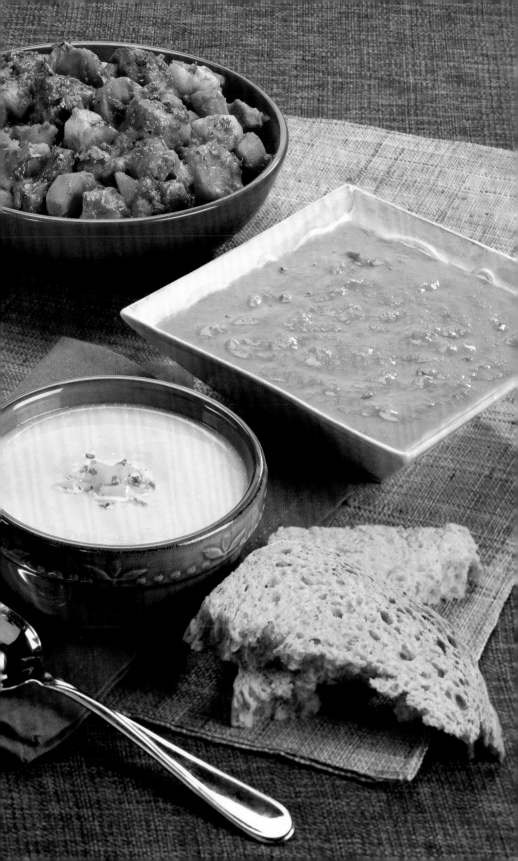

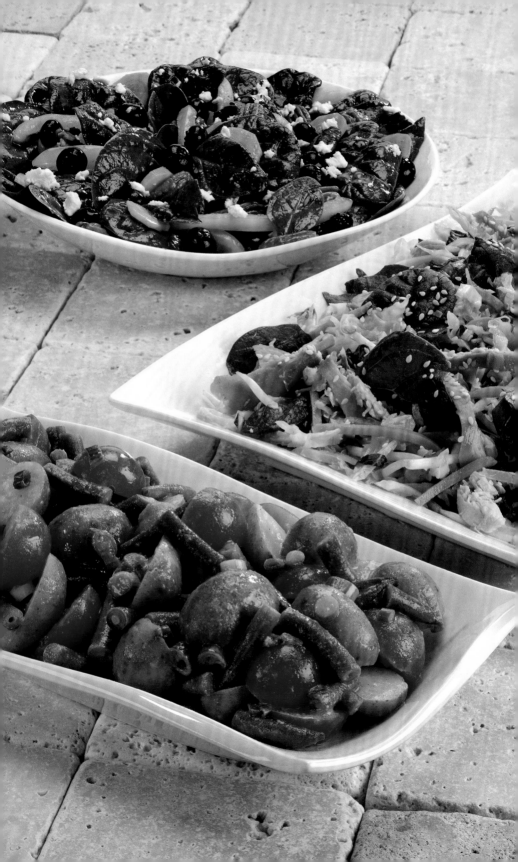

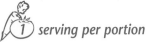

Radish Arugula Salad

The peppery flavours of arugula and radish are dressed up with sweet green apples and grated Parmesan.

Arugula, lightly packed	3 cups	750 mL
Spring mix lettuce, lightly packed	3 cups	750 mL
Chopped unpeeled tart apple	3/4 cup	175 mL
(such as Granny Smith)		
Thinly sliced radish	3/4 cup	175 mL
Buttermilk	1/3 cup	75 mL
Mayonnaise	1 tbsp.	15 mL
Dijon mustard	1/2 tsp.	2 mL
Lemon juice	1/2 tsp.	2 mL
Poppy seeds	1/2 tsp.	2 mL
Granulated sugar	1/4 tsp.	1 mL
Salt	1/8 tsp.	0.5 mL
Coarsely ground pepper	1/8 tsp.	0.5 mL
Grated Parmesan cheese	1/4 cup	60 mL

Put first 4 ingredients into large bowl. Toss.

Whisk next 8 ingredients in small bowl. Drizzle over arugula mixture.

Add cheese. Toss. Makes about 8 cups (2 L). Serves 4.

1 serving: 80 Calories; 4.5 g Total Fat (0 g Mono, 0 g Poly, 1 g Sat); 5 mg Cholesterol; 7 g Carbohydrate; 1 g Fibre; 3 g Protein; 170 mg Sodium

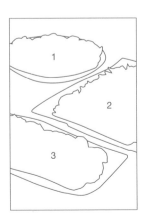

1. Rainbow Spinach Salad, page 38
2. Asian Chicken Salad, page 39
3. Green Bean Potato Salad, page 40

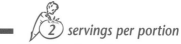

Rainbow Spinach Salad

This colourful and inviting salad packs in a splendid array of flavours and textures, all topped off with a sprinkle of feta.

Fresh spinach leaves, lightly packed	4 cups	1 L
Fresh (or frozen, thawed) blueberries	1 cup	250 mL
Thinly sliced carrot	1 cup	250 mL
Thinly sliced yellow pepper	1 cup	250 mL
Pecan halves, toasted (see Tip, below)	1/2 cup	125 mL
Cooking oil	2 tbsp.	30 mL
White wine vinegar	2 tbsp.	30 mL
Liquid honey	1 tbsp.	15 mL
Salt	1/4 tsp.	1 mL
Crumbled feta cheese	1/4 cup	60 mL

Put first 5 ingredients into large bowl. Toss.

Whisk next 4 ingredients in small bowl. Drizzle over spinach mixture. Toss.

Scatter cheese over top. Makes about 8 cups (2 L). Serves 4.

1 serving: 240 Calories; 20 g Total Fat (10 g Mono, 5 g Poly, 3 g Sat); 10 mg Cholesterol; 16 g Carbohydrate; 3 g Fibre; 4 g Protein; 260 mg Sodium

Pictured on page 36.

 When toasting nuts, seeds or coconut, cooking times will vary for each type of nut—so never toast them together. For small amounts, place ingredient in an ungreased shallow frying pan. Heat on medium for 3 to 5 minutes, stirring often, until golden. For larger amounts, spread ingredient evenly in an ungreased shallow pan. Bake in a 350°F (175°C) oven for 5 to 10 minutes, stirring or shaking often, until golden.

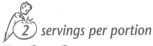

Asian Chicken Salad

A colourful and crunchy combination of fresh ingredients, with tender pieces
of marinated chicken and a gingery soy dressing to complete the experience.
A nice, light meal for a warm evening.

Soy sauce	3 tbsp.	45 mL
Brown sugar, packed	2 tsp.	10 mL
Ground ginger	1/8 tsp.	0.5 mL
Boneless, skinless chicken breast halves	2	2
(4 – 6 oz., 113 – 170 g, each)		
Rice vinegar	1/3 cup	75 mL
Sesame oil (for flavour)	3 tbsp.	45 mL
Smooth peanut butter	2 tbsp.	30 mL
Soy sauce	2 tbsp.	30 mL
Brown sugar, packed	1 tbsp.	15 mL
Chili paste (sambal oelek)	1/2 tsp.	2 mL
Garlic powder	1/4 tsp.	1 mL
Ground ginger	1/4 tsp.	1 mL
Shredded savoy cabbage, lightly packed	4 cups	1 L
Fresh bean sprouts	2 cups	500 mL
Fresh spinach leaves, lightly packed	1 cup	250 mL
Thinly sliced bok choy	1 cup	250 mL
Julienned carrot (see Tip, page 15)	1/2 cup	125 mL
Roasted sesame seeds	2 tbsp.	30 mL

Combine first 3 ingredients in shallow bowl. Add chicken. Turn until
coated. Marinate, covered, in refrigerator for 1 hour. Transfer chicken to
greased baking sheet with sides. Discard any remaining soy sauce mixture.
Broil on centre rack in oven for about 8 minutes per side until internal
temperature reaches 170°F (77°C). Transfer to cutting board. Let stand until
cool enough to handle. Slice thinly.

Whisk next 8 ingredients in extra-large bowl until smooth.

Add next 5 ingredients and chicken. Toss until coated.

Sprinkle with sesame seeds. Makes about 10 cups (2.5 L). Serves 6.

1 serving: 180 Calories; 10 g Total Fat (3 g Mono, 3 g Poly, 2 g Sat); 20 mg Cholesterol;
10 g Carbohydrate; 2 g Fibre; 13 g Protein; 780 mg Sodium

Pictured on page 36.

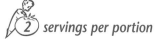
Green Bean Potato Salad

Not your usual potato salad, with plenty of colour from tomatoes and green beans and a tangy dressing to round out the flavours. A perfect companion for grilled meats.

Red baby potatoes, halved	1 lb.	454 g
Salt	1 tsp.	5 mL
Chopped fresh (or frozen) whole green beans	1 1/2 cups	375 mL
Lemon juice	3 tbsp.	45 mL
Olive (or cooking) oil	3 tbsp.	45 mL
Dijon mustard	2 tbsp.	30 mL
Liquid honey	1 tsp.	5 mL
Salt	1/4 tsp.	1 mL
Pepper	1/8 tsp.	0.5 mL
Halved cherry tomatoes	1 cup	250 mL
Sliced green onion	1/4 cup	60 mL

Pour water into large saucepan until about 1 inch (2.5 cm) deep. Add potato and first amount of salt. Cover. Bring to a boil. Reduce heat to medium. Boil gently for 10 minutes.

Add beans. Boil gently for about 4 minutes until potatoes are tender. Drain. Let stand for 30 minutes.

Whisk next 6 ingredients in large bowl.

Add tomatoes, green onion and potato mixture. Stir. Makes about 6 cups (1.5 L). Serves 6.

1 serving: 140 Calories; 7 g Total Fat (4.5 g Mono, 1 g Poly, 1 g Sat); 0 mg Cholesterol; 17 g Carbohydrate; 3 g Fibre; 2 g Protein; 550 mg Sodium

Pictured on page 36.

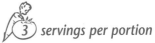

Mexican Corn Chowder

Sweet and mildly spicy chowder with crisp corn and lots of potatoes.
Serve this colourful and homey chowder with a side salad for lunch.

Bacon slices, chopped	4	4
Chopped celery	1 cup	250 mL
Chopped onion	1 cup	250 mL
Garlic cloves, minced	2	2
(or 1/2 tsp., 2 mL, powder)		
All-purpose flour	2 tbsp.	30 mL
Prepared chicken (or vegetable) broth	3 cups	750 mL
Diced unpeeled red potato	2 cups	500 mL
Fresh (or frozen) kernel corn	2 cups	500 mL
Jar of roasted red peppers,	12 oz.	340 mL
drained and chopped		
Ground cumin	1/2 tsp.	2 mL
Salt	1/4 tsp.	1 mL
Pepper	1/4 tsp.	1 mL
Milk	1/2 cup	125 mL
Lime juice	1 tbsp.	15 mL

Cook bacon in large saucepan on medium until almost crisp. Drain and discard all but 2 tsp. (10 mL) drippings.

Add next 3 ingredients. Cook for about 10 minutes, stirring often, until onion starts to brown.

Add flour. Heat and stir for 1 minute. Slowly add broth, stirring constantly until smooth. Heat and stir until boiling and thickened.

Add next 6 ingredients. Stir. Bring to a boil. Reduce heat to medium-low. Simmer, partially covered, for about 25 minutes, stirring often, until potato is tender.

Add milk and lime juice. Stir. Cook for about 2 minutes, stirring occasionally, until heated through. Makes 7 cups (1.75 L). Serves 4.

1 serving: 260 Calories; 7 g Total Fat (2.5 g Mono, 0.5 g Poly, 2 g Sat); 15 mg Cholesterol; 40 g Carbohydrate; 5 g Fibre; 9 g Protein; 790 mg Sodium

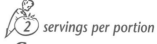

Pea and Lettuce Soup

Lovely salad flavours—in a refreshing soup! Simple ingredients come together in this exceptional chilled soup. A great method for using up those bountiful summer peas.

Cooking oil	2 tsp.	10 mL
Chopped onion	1 cup	250 mL
Frozen peas	5 cups	1.25 L
Shredded romaine lettuce, lightly packed	2 cups	500 mL
Pepper	1/4 tsp.	1 mL
Prepared vegetable broth	4 cups	1 L
Half-and-half cream	1/4 cup	60 mL
Chopped fresh chives (or green onion)	1 tbsp.	15 mL

Heat cooking oil in large saucepan on medium. Add onion. Cook for about 5 minutes, stirring often, until softened.

Add next 3 ingredients. Cook for about 8 minutes, stirring occasionally, until peas are tender and lettuce is wilted.

Add broth. Stir. Bring to a boil. Reduce heat to medium-low. Simmer, uncovered, for 5 minutes. Remove from heat. Process with hand blender, or in blender in batches, until almost smooth (see Safety Tip).

Add cream. Stir. Chill, covered.

Sprinkle with chives. Makes about 7 cups (1.75 L). Serves 6.

1 serving: 140 Calories; 3.5 g Total Fat (1.5 g Mono, 0 g Poly, 1 g Sat); trace Cholesterol; 22 g Carbohydrate; 6 g Fibre; 8 g Protein; 520 mg Sodium

Safety Tip: Follow manufacturer's instructions for processing hot liquids.

 To make hard-cooked eggs, place eggs in a single layer in a saucepan. Add cold water until it's about 1 inch (2.5 cm) above the eggs. Bring to a boil, covered. Reduce heat to medium-low. Simmer for 10 minutes. Drain. Cover the eggs with cold water. Change the water each time it warms until the eggs are cool enough to handle. Remove the shells.

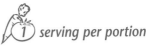

Potato Lentil Soup

Hearty and comforting, this potato soup is given bistro-style flair with the addition of goat cheese. A recipe that can't be beat.

Bacon slices, chopped	4	4
Chopped onion	1 cup	250 mL
Diced carrot	1 cup	250 mL
Diced celery rib, with leaves	1/2 cup	125 mL
Prepared chicken broth	6 cups	1.5 L
Can of lentils, rinsed and drained	19 oz.	540 mL
Baby potatoes, quartered	1/2 lb.	225 g
Bay leaves	2	2
Sprigs of fresh thyme	2	2
(or 1/8 tsp., 0.5 mL, dried)		
Chopped fresh parsley	1/4 cup	60 mL
Goat (chèvre) cheese, cut up	4 1/2 oz.	125 g

Cook bacon in Dutch oven on medium until almost crisp. Drain and discard all but 2 tsp. (10 mL) drippings.

Add next 3 ingredients. Cook for about 10 minutes, stirring often, until onion is softened.

Add next 5 ingredients. Heat and stir, scraping any brown bits from bottom of pot, until boiling. Reduce heat to medium-low. Simmer, covered, for about 25 minutes until potato is tender. Remove and discard bay leaves and thyme sprigs.

Add parsley. Stir.

Scatter cheese over individual servings. Makes about 9 cups (2.25 L). Serves 6.

1 serving: 210 Calories; 8 g Total Fat (2.5 g Mono, 0.5 g Poly, 4.5 g Sat); 15 mg Cholesterol; 22 g Carbohydrate; 6 g Fibre; 11 g Protein; 790 mg Sodium

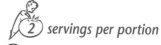

Golden Velvet Soup

Remarkably sophisticated flavours from a rather simple recipe. Smooth, velvety texture with the delicious tastes of sweet pear and root vegetables. Even the kids will enjoy this elegant dish.

Can of pear halves in juice (with juice)	28 oz.	796 mL
Prepared vegetable broth	3 cups	750 mL
Water	1 cup	250 mL
Chopped acorn squash (see Tip, page 33)	2 cups	500 mL
Chopped yellow turnip (rutabaga)	2 cups	500 mL
Chopped onion	1 cup	250 mL
Chopped parsnip	1 cup	250 mL
Chopped peeled potato	1 cup	250 mL

Combine all 8 ingredients in Dutch oven. Bring to a boil. Reduce heat to medium-low. Simmer, covered, for about 1 hour until vegetables are tender. Carefully process with hand blender, or in blender in batches, until smooth (see Safety Tip). Makes about 10 cups (2.5 L). Serves 6.

1 serving: 140 Calories; 0 g Total Fat (0 g Mono, 0 g Poly, 0 g Sat); 0 mg Cholesterol; 34 g Carbohydrate; 4 g Fibre; 2 g Protein; 320 mg Sodium

Safety Tip: Follow manufacturer's instructions for processing hot liquids.

 servings per portion

Bacon and Egg Tossed Salad

Bacon and eggs aren't just for breakfast anymore. This recipe features them as sensational salad toppings. Also a delightful option for brunch or lunch.

Cut or torn iceberg lettuce, lightly packed	3 cups	750 mL
Cut or torn romaine lettuce, lightly packed	3 cups	750 mL
Chopped Roma (plum) tomato	1 cup	250 mL
Grated sharp Cheddar cheese	1/2 cup	125 mL
Unseasoned croutons	1/2 cup	125 mL
Bacon slices, cooked crisp and crumbled	6	6
Large hard-cooked eggs, chopped (see Tip, page 42)	2	2
Sliced green onion	3 tbsp.	45 mL

(continued on next page)

White vinegar	3 tbsp.	45 mL
Cooking oil	2 tbsp.	30 mL
Dijon mustard	1 tsp.	5 mL
Granulated sugar	1 tsp.	5 mL
Salt	1/4 tsp.	1 mL
Pepper	1/8 tsp.	0.5 mL

Put first 8 ingredients into large bowl. Toss.

Whisk remaining 6 ingredients in small bowl. Drizzle over lettuce mixture. Toss. Makes about 8 cups (2 L). Serves 4.

1 serving: 230 Calories; 17 g Total Fat (8 g Mono, 3 g Poly, 4.5 g Sat); 125 mg Cholesterol; 10 g Carbohydrate; 2 g Fibre; 11 g Protein; 360 mg Sodium

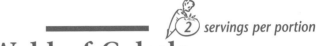 *servings per portion*

Waldorf Coleslaw

A welcome departure from your everyday coleslaw—fresh, crunchy coleslaw with pieces of sweet apple, jicama and toasted walnuts.

Mayonnaise	1/3 cup	75 mL
Lemon juice	2 tbsp.	30 mL
Granulated sugar	1 tbsp.	15 mL
Celery seed	1/4 tsp.	1 mL
Salt, sprinkle		

Coleslaw mix	4 cups	1 L
Diced unpeeled cooking apple (such as McIntosh)	1 cup	250 mL
Diced peeled jicama	1/2 cup	125 mL
Thinly sliced celery	1/2 cup	125 mL
Chopped walnuts, toasted (see Tip, page 38)	1/3 cup	75 mL

Stir first 5 ingredients in large bowl until sugar is dissolved.

Add remaining 5 ingredients. Stir well. Makes about 5 cups (1.25 L). Serves 4.

1 serving: 260 Calories; 22 g Total Fat (1 g Mono, 5 g Poly, 2.5 g Sat); 5 mg Cholesterol; 15 g Carbohydrate; 4 g Fibre; 3 g Protein; 125 mg Sodium

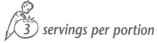

Roasted Cauliflower Soup

A bowl of thick and satisfying cauliflower soup is an excellent method for adding more vegetables to your daily meal plan. This lovely autumn soup adds a warming touch of curry.

Cooking oil	2 tbsp.	30 mL
Curry powder	1 tsp.	5 mL
Granulated sugar	1/2 tsp.	2 mL
Turmeric	1/2 tsp.	2 mL
Salt	1/4 tsp.	1 mL
Pepper	1/4 tsp.	1 mL
Cauliflower florets	4 cups	1 L
Chopped peeled potato	2 cups	500 mL
(3/4 inch, 2 cm, pieces)		
Chopped onion	1 cup	250 mL
Garlic cloves	2	2
Prepared vegetable broth	4 cups	1 L
Milk	1/2 cup	125 mL

Combine first 6 ingredients in large bowl.

Add next 4 ingredients. Toss until coated. Arrange in single layer on large greased baking sheet with sides. Cook in 400°F (200°C) oven for about 25 minutes until cauliflower is tender and golden. Transfer to large saucepan.

Add broth. Stir. Bring to a boil. Reduce heat to medium-low. Simmer, partially covered, for 20 minutes, stirring occasionally, to blend flavours.

Add milk. Stir. Carefully process with hand blender, or in blender in batches, until smooth (see Safety Tip). Makes about 7 cups (1.75 L). Serves 4.

1 serving: 180 Calories; 7 g Total Fat (4 g Mono, 2 g Poly, 1 g Sat); 0 mg Cholesterol; 26 g Carbohydrate; 4 g Fibre; 6 g Protein; 750 mg Sodium

Safety Tip: Follow manufacturer's instructions for processing hot liquids.

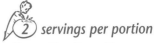
Sweet Potato Avocado Salad

This unique potato salad features sweet potato as a welcome addition.
Avocado, tomato, cilantro and a tangy dressing add extra punch to this
colourful dish.

Cubed peeled orange-fleshed sweet potato (3/4 inch, 2 cm, pieces)	3 cups	750 mL
Cubed peeled potato (1/2 inch, 12 mm, pieces)	1 1/2 cups	375 mL
Cooking oil	1 tbsp.	15 mL
Chili powder	1/2 tsp.	2 mL
Salt	1/4 tsp.	1 mL
Pepper	1/4 tsp.	1 mL
Sour cream	1/2 cup	125 mL
Lime juice	2 tbsp.	30 mL
Finely chopped fresh jalapeño pepper (see Tip, below)	4 tsp.	20 mL
Chopped fresh cilantro (or parsley)	1 tbsp.	15 mL
Salt	1/4 tsp.	1 mL
Chopped avocado	1 cup	250 mL
Halved grape tomatoes	1 cup	250 mL
Grated Mexican cheese blend	1/2 cup	125 mL
Chopped green onion	2 tbsp.	30 mL

Toss first 6 ingredients in large bowl until coated. Arrange in single layer on greased baking sheet with sides. Cook in 375°F (190°C) oven for about 30 minutes until tender. Return to large bowl. Cool.

Combine next 5 ingredients in small bowl. Add to sweet potato mixture. Stir.

Add remaining 4 ingredients. Stir. Makes about 6 cups (1.5 L). Serves 6.

1 serving: 180 Calories; 11 g Total Fat (4 g Mono, 1 g Poly, 4.5 g Sat); 15 mg Cholesterol; 17 g Carbohydrate; 3 g Fibre; 4 g Protein; 260 mg Sodium

 tip   Hot peppers contain capsaicin in the seeds and ribs. Removing the seeds and ribs will reduce the heat. Wear rubber gloves when handling hot peppers and avoid touching your eyes. Wash your hands well afterwards.

Rhubarb Streusel Muffins

Rhubarb, though often thought of as a fruit, is actually a vegetable. Here it's packed into tender muffins with a sweet streusel topping for a delicious dose of veggie power.

All-purpose flour	1 3/4 cup	425 mL
Brown sugar, packed	1 cup	250 mL
Baking powder	1 tsp.	5 mL
Baking soda	1 tsp.	5 mL
Salt	1/2 tsp.	2 mL
Large egg, fork-beaten	1	1
Buttermilk (or soured milk, see Tip, page 60)	2/3 cup	150 mL
Cooking oil	1/3 cup	75 mL
Frozen concentrated orange juice, thawed	2 tbsp.	30 mL
Vanilla extract	1 tsp.	5 mL
Finely diced frozen rhubarb, thawed	1 1/4 cups	300 mL
Chopped walnuts	1/2 cup	125 mL
Finely chopped walnuts	1/4 cup	60 mL
All-purpose flour	3 tbsp.	45 mL
Brown sugar, packed	3 tbsp.	45 mL
Frozen concentrated orange juice, thawed	2 tsp.	10 mL

Combine first 5 ingredients in large bowl. Make a well in centre.

Combine next 5 ingredients in medium bowl. Add to well.

Add rhubarb and first amount of walnuts. Stir until just moistened. Fill 12 greased muffin cups 3/4 full.

Stir remaining 4 ingredients in small bowl until mixture resembles coarse crumbs. Sprinkle over top. Bake in 375°F (190°C) oven for about 20 minutes until wooden pick inserted in centre of muffin comes out clean. Let stand in pan for 5 minutes before removing to wire rack to cool. Makes 12 muffins.

1 muffin: 280 Calories; 11 g Total Fat (4.5 g Mono, 5 g Poly, 1 g Sat); 10 mg Cholesterol; 41 g Carbohydrate; 1 g Fibre; 4 g Protein; 230 mg Sodium

Pictured on page 18.

Chocolate Veggie Bread

Kohlrabi and carrot are paired up with chocolate in this moist, decadent bread.
Accents of cinnamon and orange zest round out the flavours.

All-purpose flour	1 1/2 cups	375 mL
Granulated sugar	1/2 cup	125 mL
Cocoa, sifted if lumpy	1/3 cup	75 mL
Baking powder	2 tsp.	10 mL
Baking soda	1/2 tsp.	2 mL
Ground cinnamon	1/2 tsp.	2 mL
Salt	1/8 tsp.	0.5 mL
Large eggs, fork-beaten	2	2
Grated kohlrabi	1 cup	250 mL
Buttermilk (or soured milk, see Tip, page 60)	1/2 cup	125 mL
Grated carrot	1/2 cup	125 mL
Cooking oil	2 tbsp.	30 mL
Grated orange zest	1 tsp.	5 mL
Mini semi-sweet chocolate chips	1/2 cup	125 mL

Combine first 7 ingredients in large bowl. Make a well in centre.

Combine next 6 ingredients in medium bowl. Add to well.

Add chocolate chips. Stir until just moistened. Spread in greased 9 x 5 x 3 inch (23 x 12.5 x 7.5 cm) loaf pan. Bake in 350°F (175°C) oven for about 50 minutes until wooden pick inserted in centre comes out clean. Let stand in pan for 10 minutes before removing to wire rack to cool. Cuts into 16 slices.

1 slice: 130 Calories; 4 g Total Fat (2 g Mono, 0.5 g Poly, 1.5 g Sat); 20 mg Cholesterol; 21 g Carbohydrate; 2 g Fibre; 3 g Protein; 105 mg Sodium

HELPFUL HINTS When choosing kohlrabi, select bulbs that are under 3 inches (7.5 cm) in diameter and free of cracks.

Tomato Herb Bread

Try making a BLT sandwich with the tomato baked right into the bread—how's that for inventive?

Warm water (see Tip, page 51)	1/4 cup	60 mL
Granulated sugar	1 1/2 tsp.	7 mL
Envelope of active dry yeast	1/4 oz.	8 g
(or 2 1/4 tsp., 11 mL)		
Tomato juice, room temperature	1 cup	250 mL
Cooking oil	2 tbsp.	30 mL
Tomato paste (see Tip, page 32)	2 tbsp.	30 mL
All-purpose flour	2 1/2 cups	625 mL
Whole-wheat flour	1 1/4 cups	300 mL
Dried basil	1 tsp.	5 mL
Dried oregano	1 tsp.	5 mL
Dried thyme	1/2 tsp.	2 mL
Salt	1 tsp.	5 mL
Pepper	1/4 tsp.	1 mL

Stir water and sugar in small bowl until sugar is dissolved. Sprinkle yeast over top. Let stand for 10 minutes. Stir until yeast is dissolved.

Add next 3 ingredients. Stir.

Combine next 7 ingredients in large bowl. Make a well in centre. Add yeast mixture. Mix until soft dough forms. Turn out dough onto lightly floured surface. Knead for 5 to 10 minutes until smooth and elastic. Place in greased extra-large bowl, turning once to grease top. Cover with greased waxed paper and tea towel. Let stand in oven with light on and door closed for about 1 hour until doubled in bulk. Punch dough down. Turn out onto lightly floured surface. Knead for about 1 minute until smooth. Shape into loaf. Place in greased 9 x 5 x 3 inch (23 x 12.5 x 7.5 cm) loaf pan. Cover with greased waxed paper and tea towel. Let stand in oven with light on and door closed for about 1 hour until doubled in size. Bake in 375°F (190°C) oven for about 30 minutes until golden and hollow sounding when tapped. Remove bread from pan and place on wire rack to cool. Cuts into 16 slices.

1 slice: 130 Calories; 2 g Total Fat (1 g Mono, 0.5 g Poly, 0 g Sat); 0 mg Cholesterol; 23 g Carbohydrate; 2 g Fibre; 4 g Protein; 200 mg Sodium

Pictured on page 35.

Sesame Cabbage Loaf

What a tasty and unexpected method for using up leftover cabbage! The strands of red cabbage give the appearance of blueberries in this soft wheat loaf. Serve toasted with a bowl of soup.

All-purpose flour	1 cup	250 mL
Whole-wheat flour	1 cup	250 mL
Roasted sesame seeds	1/4 cup	60 mL
Baking powder	2 tsp.	10 mL
Baking soda	1/2 tsp.	2 mL
Salt	1/2 tsp.	2 mL
Dry mustard	1/4 tsp.	1 mL
Ground ginger	1/4 tsp.	1 mL
Large egg, fork-beaten	1	1
Plain yogurt	1/2 cup	125 mL
Prepared chicken broth	1/2 cup	125 mL
Cooking oil	1/4 cup	60 mL
Granulated sugar	1 tbsp.	15 mL
Shredded red cabbage, lightly packed	1 cup	250 mL

Combine first 8 ingredients in large bowl. Make a well in centre.

Combine next 5 ingredients in medium bowl. Add to well.

Add cabbage. Stir until just moistened. Spread in greased 9 x 5 x 3 inch (23 x 12.5 x 7.5 cm) loaf pan. Bake in 350°F (175°C) oven for about 50 minutes until wooden pick inserted in centre comes out clean. Let stand in pan for 10 minutes before removing to wire rack to cool. Cuts into 16 slices.

1 slice: 110 Calories; 5 g Total Fat (2.5 g Mono, 1.5 g Poly, 0.5 g Sat); 10 mg Cholesterol; 14 g Carbohydrate; 2 g Fibre; 3 g Protein; 190 mg Sodium

 tip When using yeast, it is important for the liquid to be at the correct temperature. If the liquid is too cool, the yeast will not activate properly. If the liquid is too hot, the yeast will be destroyed. For best results, follow the recommended temperatures as instructed on the package.

Turnip Ginger Muffins

Soft, sweet muffins with a moist texture and a hint of ginger. No one will ever guess that turnip is the secret ingredient!

All-purpose flour	1 1/2 cups	375 mL
Brown sugar, packed	3/4 cup	175 mL
Quick-cooking rolled oats	1/2 cup	125 mL
Baking powder	1 tsp.	5 mL
Ground ginger	1 tsp.	5 mL
Baking soda	1/2 tsp.	2 mL
Salt	1/2 tsp.	2 mL
Large eggs, fork-beaten	2	2
Buttermilk (or soured milk, see Tip, page 60)	3/4 cup	175 mL
Cooking oil	1/3 cup	75 mL
Vanilla extract	1 tsp.	5 mL
Grated purple-topped turnip	2 cups	500 mL

Combine first 7 ingredients in large bowl. Make a well in centre.

Combine next 4 ingredients in medium bowl. Add to well.

Add turnip. Stir until just moistened. Fill 12 greased muffin cups 3/4 full. Bake in 375°F (190°C) oven for about 20 minutes until wooden pick inserted in centre of muffin comes out clean. Let stand in pan for 5 minutes before removing to wire rack to cool. Makes 12 muffins.

1 muffin: 200 Calories; 7 g Total Fat (4 g Mono, 2 g Poly, 1 g Sat); 25 mg Cholesterol; 30 g Carbohydrate; 1 g Fibre; 4 g Protein; 190 mg Sodium

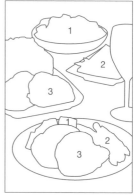

1. Spiced Sweet Potatoes, page 134
2. Grilled Asparagus, page 134
3. Rhubarb-stuffed Pork, page 100

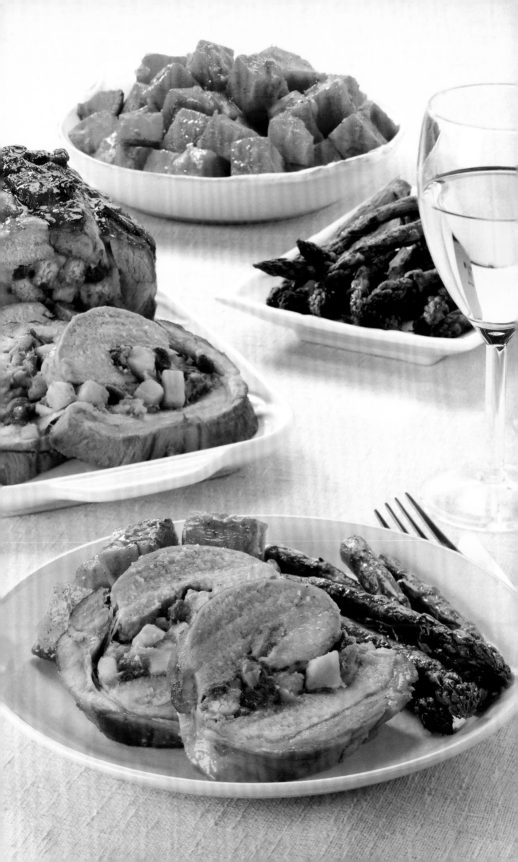

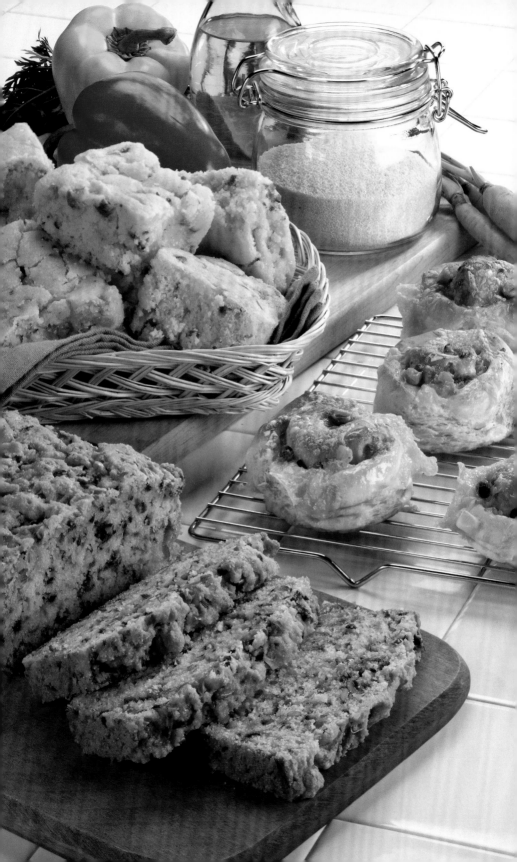

Zucchini Onion Biscuits

These versatile biscuits are packed with flavourful onion and a nice hint of Parmesan—almost like a cross between green onion cakes and cheese buns.

All-purpose flour	2 cups	500 mL
Grated Parmesan cheese	1/4 cup	60 mL
Baking powder	4 tsp.	20 mL
Granulated sugar	1 tsp.	5 mL
Italian seasoning	1/2 tsp.	2 mL
Salt	1/2 tsp.	2 mL
Pepper	1/4 tsp.	1 mL
Cold butter (or hard margarine), cut up	1/3 cup	75 mL
Grated zucchini (with peel)	3/4 cup	175 mL
Plain yogurt	3/4 cup	175 mL
Thinly sliced green onion	1/2 cup	125 mL
Milk	1/4 cup	60 mL

Combine first 7 ingredients in large bowl. Cut in butter until mixture resembles coarse crumbs. Make a well in centre.

Combine remaining 4 ingredients in small bowl. Add to well. Stir until just moistened. Drop, using 1/4 cup (60 mL) for each, about 2 inches (5 cm) apart on greased baking sheet. Bake in 400°F (200°C) oven for about 15 minutes until golden. Let stand on baking sheet for 5 minutes before removing to wire rack to cool. Makes about 18 biscuits.

1 biscuit: 100 Calories; 4.5 g Total Fat (1 g Mono, 0 g Poly, 2.5 g Sat); 10 mg Cholesterol; 12 g Carbohydrate; trace Fibre; 3 g Protein; 170 mg Sodium

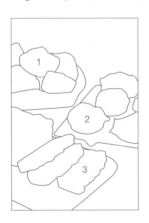

1. Sweet Chipotle Cornbread, page 56
2. Veggie Cheddar Spirals, page 57
3. Garden Rainbow Loaf, page 59

Sweet Chipotle Cornbread

*This colourful cornbread is both sweet and spicy. You'll find plenty of veggies
here, and even a bit of fruit!*

All-purpose flour	1 1/2 cups	375 mL
Yellow cornmeal	1 cup	250 mL
Baking powder	2 tsp.	10 mL
Baking soda	1/2 tsp.	2 mL
Salt	1/2 tsp.	2 mL
Large eggs, fork-beaten	2	2
Buttermilk (or soured milk, see Tip, page 60)	1 cup	250 mL
Cooking oil	1/3 cup	75 mL
Liquid honey	1/4 cup	60 mL
Finely chopped chipotle peppers in adobo sauce (see Tip, below)	1 tbsp.	15 mL
Chopped dried apricot	1/2 cup	125 mL
Chopped green onion	1/2 cup	125 mL
Finely chopped red pepper	1/2 cup	125 mL
Frozen kernel corn, thawed	1/2 cup	125 mL

Combine first 5 ingredients in large bowl. Make a well in centre.

Combine next 5 ingredients in medium bowl. Add to well.

Add remaining 4 ingredients. Stir until just moistened. Spread in greased
9 x 9 inch (23 x 23 cm) pan. Bake in 350°F (175°C) oven for about
30 minutes until wooden pick inserted in centre comes out clean. Let stand
in pan for 10 minutes before removing to wire rack to cool. Cuts into
9 pieces.

*1 piece: 280 Calories; 11 g Total Fat (5 g Mono, 2.5 g Poly, 1 g Sat); 30 mg Cholesterol;
44 g Carbohydrate; 2 g Fibre; 6 g Protein; 280 mg Sodium*

Pictured on page 54.

 tip   Chipotle chili peppers are smoked jalapeño peppers. Be sure to wash
your hands after handling. To store any leftover chipotle peppers,
divide into recipe-friendly portions and freeze, with sauce, in airtight
containers for up to one year.

Veggie Cheddar Spirals

Perfect for an after-school snack or a portable lunch for the kids. Features great flavours that are similar to pizza buns.

Bacon slices, chopped	2	2
Chopped onion	3/4 cup	175 mL
All-purpose flour	1 tbsp.	15 mL
Frozen pea and carrot mix, thawed	1/2 cup	125 mL
Grated medium Cheddar cheese	3/4 cup	175 mL
Frozen white bread dough, covered, thawed in refrigerator overnight	1	1
Grated medium Cheddar cheese	1/2 cup	125 mL

Cook bacon in medium frying pan on medium until crisp. Transfer with slotted spoon to paper towel–lined plate to drain. Drain and discard all but 1 tsp. (5 mL) drippings.

Add onion to same frying pan. Cook for about 5 minutes, stirring often, until softened.

Add flour. Heat and stir for 1 minute. Add pea and carrot mix and bacon. Stir. Transfer to medium bowl. Let stand for 10 minutes to cool slightly.

Add first amount of cheese. Stir.

Roll out dough to 10 x 14 inch (25 x 35 cm) rectangle. Spread bacon mixture over dough to within 1/2 inch (12 mm) of edge. Roll up, jelly roll-style, from long side. Pinch seam against roll to seal. Cut into 12 slices using serrated knife. Arrange, cut-side up, in greased 9 x 13 inch (23 x 33 cm) pan. Cover with greased waxed paper and tea towel. Let stand in oven with light on and door closed for about 1 hour until doubled in size.

Sprinkle with second amount of cheese. Bake on centre rack in 375°F (190°C) oven for about 25 minutes until golden. Let stand on baking sheet for 5 minutes before removing to wire rack to cool. Makes 12 spirals.

1 spiral: 170 Calories; 6 g Total Fat (1.5 g Mono, 0.5 g Poly, 2.5 g Sat); 10 mg Cholesterol; 22 g Carbohydrate; 1 g Fibre; 7 g Protein; 290 mg Sodium

Pictured on page 54.

Pumpkin Cranberry Buns

Granted, pumpkin may technically be a fruit, but there's no denying that it's healthy! These moist, chewy dinner rolls boast an attractive orange colour from pumpkin accompanied by lovely notes of cinnamon.

All-purpose flour	3 cups	750 mL
Envelope of instant yeast (or 2 1/4 tsp., 11 mL)	1/4 oz.	8 g
Salt	1 tsp.	5 mL
Ground cinnamon	1/2 tsp.	2 mL
Milk	3/4 cup	175 mL
Canned pure pumpkin (no spices), see Tip, page 23	1/2 cup	125 mL
Granulated sugar	2 tbsp.	30 mL
Butter (or hard margarine)	1 tbsp.	15 mL
Large egg, fork-beaten	1	1
Dried cranberries	3/4 cup	175 mL
All-purpose flour, approximately	1 tbsp.	15 mL
Butter (or hard margarine), melted	1 tbsp.	15 mL

Combine first 4 ingredients in large bowl. Make a well in centre.

Combine next 4 ingredients in small saucepan. Heat and stir on medium until very warm (see Tip, page 51). Add to well. Stir.

Add egg. Mix until soft dough forms.

Add cranberries. Mix. Turn out onto lightly floured surface.

Knead for 5 to 10 minutes until smooth and elastic, adding second amount of flour, 1 tbsp. (15 mL) at a time, if necessary, to prevent sticking. Place in greased extra-large bowl, turning once to grease top. Cover with greased waxed paper and tea towel. Let stand in oven with light on and door closed for about 1 hour until doubled in bulk. Punch dough down. Turn out onto lightly floured surface. Divide into 12 portions. Roll into balls. Arrange in greased 9 x 13 inch (23 x 33 cm) pan. Cover with greased waxed paper and tea towel. Let stand in oven with light on and door closed for about 45 minutes until doubled in size.

(continued on next page)

Breads

Brush with second amount of butter. Bake in 350°F (175°C) oven for about 25 minutes until golden and hollow sounding when tapped. Let stand in pan for 5 minutes before removing to wire rack to cool. Makes 12 buns.

1 bun: 180 Calories; 3 g Total Fat (0.5 g Mono, 0 g Poly, 1.5 g Sat); 15 mg Cholesterol; 34 g Carbohydrate; 2 g Fibre; 5 g Protein; 230 mg Sodium

Garden Rainbow Loaf

Find a spectrum of colour in this unique loaf. The top is orange, the interior is yellow and it's delicious all the way through.

All-purpose flour	1 1/2 cups	375 mL
Yellow cornmeal	1/2 cup	125 mL
Granulated sugar	3 tbsp.	45 mL
Baking powder	2 tsp.	10 mL
Baking soda	1/2 tsp.	2 mL
Salt	1/2 tsp.	2 mL
Large eggs, fork-beaten	2	2
Cooking oil	1/2 cup	125 mL
Sour cream	1/4 cup	60 mL
Finely chopped Swiss chard, lightly packed	1/2 cup	125 mL
Finely chopped yellow pepper	1/2 cup	125 mL
Grated carrot	1/2 cup	125 mL
Grated peeled beet (see Tip, page 61)	1/2 cup	125 mL
Salted, roasted sunflower seeds	1/4 cup	60 mL
Grated lime zest	3/4 tsp.	4 mL

Combine first 6 ingredients in large bowl. Make a well in centre.

·Combine next 3 ingredients in medium bowl. Add to well.

Add remaining 6 ingredients. Stir until just moistened. Spread in greased 9 x 5 x 3 inch (23 x 12.5 x 7.5 cm) loaf pan. Bake in 350°F (175°C) oven for about 45 minutes until wooden pick inserted in centre comes out clean. Let stand in pan for 10 minutes before removing to wire rack to cool. Cuts into 16 slices.

1 slice: 160 Calories; 9 g Total Fat (4.5 g Mono, 2.5 g Poly, 1 g Sat); 20 mg Cholesterol; 17 g Carbohydrate; trace Fibre; 3 g Protein; 150 mg Sodium

Pictured on page 54.

Spinach Pakora Muffins

Savoury spinach and onion muffins get a touch of Indian flair with mild curry and sweet currants. They're great with a bowl of soup.

All-purpose flour	2 cups	500 mL
Baking powder	1 tbsp.	15 mL
Curry powder	2 tsp.	10 mL
Salt	1/2 tsp.	2 mL
Large egg, fork-beaten	1	1
Box of frozen chopped spinach, thawed and squeezed dry	10 oz.	300 g
Buttermilk (or soured milk, see Tip, below)	1 cup	250 mL
Grated carrot	1 cup	250 mL
Sliced green onion	1/2 cup	125 mL
Cooking oil	1/3 cup	75 mL
Crumbled feta cheese	1/2 cup	125 mL
Currants	1/2 cup	125 mL

Combine first 4 ingredients in large bowl. Make a well in centre.

Combine next 6 ingredients in medium bowl. Add to well.

Add cheese and currants. Stir until just moistened. Fill 12 greased muffin cups full. Bake in 375°F (190°C) oven for about 22 minutes until wooden pick inserted in centre of muffin comes out clean. Let stand in pan for 5 minutes before removing to wire rack to cool. Makes 12 muffins.

1 muffin: 180 Calories; 8 g Total Fat (4 g Mono, 2 g Poly, 1.5 g Sat); 20 mg Cholesterol; 21 g Carbohydrate; 2 g Fibre; 5 g Protein; 280 mg Sodium

 tip To make soured milk, measure 1 tbsp. (15 mL) white vinegar or lemon juice into a 1 cup (250 mL) liquid measure. Add enough milk to make 1 cup (250 mL). Stir. Let stand for 1 minute.

Mushroom Focaccia

Inviting focaccia wedges with lovely complementary flavours of mushroom, caramelized onion, thyme and Swiss cheese. Simple yet delicious.

Cooking oil	1 tsp.	5 mL
Thinly sliced fresh white mushrooms	2 cups	500 mL
Thinly sliced onion	1/2 cup	125 mL
Dried thyme	1/4 tsp.	1 mL
Garlic powder	1/8 tsp.	0.5 mL
Salt	1/8 tsp.	0.5 mL
Frozen whole-wheat bread dough, covered, thawed in refrigerator overnight	1	1
Grated Swiss cheese	1/3 cup	75 mL

Heat cooking oil in large frying pan on medium-high. Add next 5 ingredients. Cook for about 5 minutes, stirring occasionally, until liquid is evaporated and mushrooms start to brown. Cool.

Press dough into greased 9 x 13 inch (23 x 33 cm) pan. Cover with greased waxed paper and tea towel. Let stand in oven with light on and door closed for about 45 minutes until doubled in size. Poke indentations on surface of dough with fingers.

Sprinkle with cheese. Scatter mushroom mixture over top. Bake in 400°F (200°C) oven for about 20 minutes until edges are golden. Let stand in pan for 5 minutes. Cut into 6 squares. Cut each square in half diagonally. Makes 12 wedges.

1 wedge: 130 Calories; 2.5 g Total Fat (0.5 g Mono, 0.5 g Poly, 0.5 g Sat); trace Cholesterol; 21 g Carbohydrate; 1 g Fibre; 5 g Protein; 230 mg Sodium

 tip Don't get caught red-handed! Wear rubber gloves when handling beets.

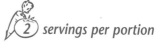

Stuffed Mexican Meatloaf

This familiar favourite is hiding something—a delicious filling of vegetables, tortilla chips and lots of tasty tex-mex flavour! Serve with salsa to make it a fiesta.

Cooking oil	2 tsp.	10 mL
Chopped onion	1/2 cup	125 mL
Chopped Swiss chard, lightly packed	3 cups	750 mL
Fresh (or frozen) kernel corn	1/2 cup	125 mL
Chili powder	1/2 tsp.	2 mL
Salt, sprinkle		
Large egg, fork-beaten	1	1
Crushed tortilla chips	1/2 cup	125 mL
Lime juice	2 tbsp.	30 mL
Taco seasoning mix, stir before measuring	2 tbsp.	30 mL
Lean ground beef	1 lb.	454 g
Grated Mexican cheese blend	1/2 cup	125 mL
Grated Mexican cheese blend	1/4 cup	60 mL

Heat cooking oil in large frying pan on medium. Add onion. Cook for about 5 minutes, stirring often, until softened.

Add next 4 ingredients. Cook for about 5 minutes, stirring occasionally, until chard is softened and liquid is evaporated.

Combine next 4 ingredients in large bowl.

Add beef. Mix well. Pat out beef mixture to 8 x 11 inch (20 x 28 cm) rectangle on large sheet of foil. Sprinkle with first amount of cheese. Spoon chard mixture lengthwise along centre of rectangle. Fold both long sides over stuffing to enclose. Pinch edges to seal. Holding foil, carefully roll meatloaf, seam-side down, onto greased wire rack set on greased baking sheet with sides. Discard foil. Cook in 350°F (175°C) oven for 45 minutes.

Sprinkle second amount of cheese over meatloaf. Cook for about 5 minutes until cheese is melted and internal temperature of beef (not stuffing) reaches 160°F (71°C). Let stand for 10 minutes. Cuts into 8 slices. Serves 4.

1 serving: 530 Calories; 32 g Total Fat (11 g Mono, 1.5 g Poly, 14 g Sat); 135 mg Cholesterol; 19 g Carbohydrate; 2 g Fibre; 33 g Protein; 850 mg Sodium

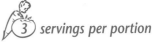

Mushroom Meatball Ragout

This thyme-scented, rich, velvety stew is brimming with mushrooms and meatballs. Just spoon over noodles or mashed potatoes to make a complete meal.

Large egg, fork-beaten	1	1
Crushed soda crackers (about 14 crackers)	1/2 cup	125 mL
Dry mustard	1/2 tsp.	2 mL
Salt	1/4 tsp.	1 mL
Pepper	1/4 tsp.	1 mL
Lean ground beef	1 lb.	454 g
Cooking oil	2 tsp.	10 mL
Small whole fresh white mushrooms	3 cups	750 mL
Baby carrots, halved	2 cups	500 mL
Chopped onion	1 cup	250 mL
Garlic cloves, minced	2	2
(or 1/2 tsp., 2 mL, powder)		
All-purpose flour	2 tbsp.	30 mL
Prepared beef broth	3 cups	750 mL
Tomato paste (see Tip, page 32)	2 tbsp.	30 mL
Granulated sugar	1 tsp.	5 mL
Dried thyme	1/2 tsp.	2 mL
Bay leaves	2	2

Combine first 5 ingredients in large bowl.

Add beef. Mix well. Roll into 1 inch (2.5 cm) balls. Arrange in single layer on greased baking sheet with sides. Broil on top rack in oven for about 8 minutes until no longer pink inside. Makes about 45 meatballs.

Heat cooking oil in large saucepan on medium. Add next 4 ingredients. Cook for about 12 minutes, stirring occasionally, until onion is softened.

Sprinkle with flour. Heat and stir for 1 minute. Add remaining 5 ingredients and meatballs. Stir. Bring to a boil. Reduce heat to medium-low. Simmer, covered, for about 30 minutes, stirring occasionally, until carrot is tender. Remove and discard bay leaves. Makes about 6 1/2 cups (1.6 L). Serves 4.

1 serving: 430 Calories; 20 g Total Fat (9 g Mono, 1.5 g Poly, 7 g Sat); 100 mg Cholesterol; 26 g Carbohydrate; 3 g Fibre; 29 g Protein; 910 mg Sodium

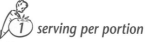

Moroccan Beef and Couscous

Spice is nice, especially in this satisfying all-in-one meal.

Cooking oil	2 tsp.	10 mL
Beef strip loin steak, cut into thin strips	3/4 lb.	340 g
Salt, sprinkle		
Pepper, sprinkle		
Cooking oil	1 tsp.	5 mL
Diced onion	1 cup	250 mL
Diced zucchini (with peel)	1/2 cup	125 mL
Finely chopped parsnip	1/4 cup	60 mL
Finely chopped purple-topped turnip	1/4 cup	60 mL
Brown sugar, packed	1 tbsp.	15 mL
Ground coriander	1/2 tsp.	2 mL
Ground cumin	1/2 tsp.	2 mL
Garlic clove, minced	1	1
(or 1/4 tsp., 1 mL, powder)		
Cayenne pepper	1/4 tsp.	1 mL
Ground cinnamon	1/4 tsp.	1 mL
Prepared vegetable broth	1 1/2 cups	375 mL
Chopped trimmed snow peas	1/2 cup	125 mL
Diced orange pepper	1/2 cup	125 mL
Red wine vinegar	1 tbsp.	15 mL
Whole-wheat couscous	1 cup	250 mL
Sliced natural almonds, toasted	2 tbsp.	30 mL
(see Tip, page 38)		

Heat first amount of cooking oil in large frying pan on medium-high. Add beef. Sprinkle with salt and pepper. Cook for about 5 minutes, stirring occasionally, until browned. Transfer to large plate. Cover to keep warm. Reduce heat to medium.

Heat second amount of cooking oil in same frying pan. Add next 10 ingredients. Cook for about 8 minutes, stirring often, until onion is softened.

Add next 4 ingredients. Stir. Bring to a boil.

(continued on next page)

64   Mains - Beef

Add couscous and beef. Stir. Remove from heat. Let stand, covered, for 5 minutes. Fluff with fork.

Add almonds. Stir. Makes about 7 1/2 cups (1.9 L). Serves 4.

1 serving: 440 Calories; 14 g Total Fat (6 g Mono, 1.5 g Poly, 3.5 g Sat); 55 mg Cholesterol; 48 g Carbohydrate; 6 g Fibre; 33 g Protein; 270 mg Sodium

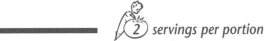 *servings per portion*

Caramelized Onion Beef Tart

These flavourful wedges are packed with sweet caramelized onion.

Butter (or hard margarine)	1/4 cup	60 mL
Sliced onion	6 cups	1.5 L
Dried thyme	1/2 tsp.	2 mL
Salt	1/8 tsp.	0.5 mL
Pepper, sprinkle		
Package of puff pastry (14 oz., 397 g), thawed according to package directions	1/2	1/2
Dijon mustard	1 tbsp.	15 mL
Finely chopped cooked roast beef	1 1/2 cups	375 mL
Grated Gruyère (or Swiss) cheese	1/2 cup	125 mL

Melt butter in large frying pan on medium. Add next 4 ingredients. Stir. Cook, covered, for about 10 minutes until onion is softened. Reduce heat to medium-low. Cook, uncovered, for about 15 minutes, stirring occasionally, until onion is caramelized.

Roll out puff pastry on lightly floured surface to 11 inch (28 cm) circle. Place on ungreased baking sheet.

Spread mustard over pastry, leaving 2 inch (5 cm) edge. Scatter beef and cheese over mustard. Spread onion mixture over cheese. Fold a section of border up and over edge of filling. Repeat with next section, allowing pastry to overlap so a fold is created. Pinch fold to seal. Repeat until pastry border is completely folded around filling. Bake in 375°F (190°C) oven for about 40 minutes until pastry is puffed and golden. Let stand for 5 minutes. Cuts into 6 wedges. Serves 6.

1 serving: 430 Calories; 29 g Total Fat (13 g Mono, 2.5 g Poly, 12 g Sat); 60 mg Cholesterol; 27 g Carbohydrate; 2 g Fibre; 14 g Protein; 250 mg Sodium

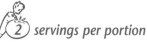

Pepper Beef Stir-fry

There's no shortage of pepper power in this vibrant stir-fry.
Serve with noodles or rice.

Prepared beef broth	1/4 cup	60 mL
Orange juice	2 tbsp.	30 mL
Soy sauce	2 tbsp.	30 mL
Sweet chili sauce	2 tbsp.	30 mL
Cornstarch	2 tsp.	10 mL
Finely grated ginger root	1 tsp.	5 mL
(or 1/4 tsp., 1 mL, ground ginger)		
Garlic clove, minced	1	1
(or 1/4 tsp., 1 mL, powder)		
Cooking oil	2 tsp.	10 mL
Beef top sirloin steak, cut into thin strips	3/4 lb.	340 g
Cooking oil	2 tsp.	10 mL
Sliced onion	1 cup	250 mL
Julienned peeled jicama (see Tip, page 15)	3/4 cup	175 mL
Thinly sliced green pepper	3/4 cup	175 mL
Thinly sliced red pepper	3/4 cup	175 mL
Thinly sliced orange pepper	3/4 cup	175 mL
Thinly sliced yellow pepper	3/4 cup	175 mL

Stir first 7 ingredients in small bowl until smooth.

Heat large frying pan or wok on medium-high until very hot. Add first amount of cooking oil. Add beef. Stir-fry for about 3 minutes until beef starts to brown. Transfer to large plate. Cover to keep warm.

Add second amount of cooking oil to same frying pan on medium-high. Add onion. Stir-fry for 2 minutes.

Add remaining 5 ingredients. Stir-fry for about 3 minutes until peppers are tender-crisp. Stir broth mixture. Add to pepper mixture. Add beef. Stir-fry for about 2 minutes until boiling and thickened. Makes about 6 cups (1.5 L). Serves 4.

1 serving: 290 Calories; 12 g Total Fat (6 g Mono, 1.5 g Poly, 3.5 g Sat); 40 mg Cholesterol; 17 g Carbohydrate; 3 g Fibre; 19 g Protein; 610 mg Sodium

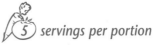

Stuffed Tuscan Squash

Tasty Mediterranean ingredients fill colourful squash halves for an impressive yet simple presentation.

Small spaghetti squash	3	3
Cooking oil	2 tsp.	10 mL
Halved fresh white mushrooms	5 cups	1.25 L
Chopped eggplant (with peel)	3 cups	750 mL
Lean ground beef	1 lb.	454 g
Chopped red onion	1 1/2 cups	375 mL
Chopped green pepper	1 cup	250 mL
Dried crushed chilies	1/2 tsp.	2 mL
Jars of marinated artichoke hearts (6 oz., 170 mL, each), drained and coarsely chopped	2	2
Chopped tomato	1/2 cup	125 mL
Sun-dried tomato pesto	1/2 cup	125 mL
Pine nuts	1/4 cup	60 mL
Grated Italian cheese blend	3/4 cup	175 mL
Chopped fresh basil	1/3 cup	75 mL

Cut squash in half lengthwise. Remove seeds. Place, cut-side down, on greased baking sheet with sides. Cook in 375°F (190°C) oven for about 40 minutes until tender. Turn squash halves cut-side up.

Heat cooking oil in large frying pan on medium-high. Add mushrooms and eggplant. Cook for about 15 minutes, stirring occasionally, until liquid is evaporated and mushrooms are browned.

Add next 4 ingredients. Scramble-fry for about 10 minutes until beef is no longer pink.

Add next 4 ingredients. Cook for about 5 minutes, stirring occasionally, until heated through. Spoon into squash halves.

Sprinkle cheese and basil over top. Broil on top rack in oven for about 5 minutes until cheese is golden. Makes 6 stuffed squash. Serves 6.

1 serving: 460 Calories; 26 g Total Fat (7 g Mono, 3.5 g Poly, 8 g Sat); 55 mg Cholesterol; 30 g Carbohydrate; 7 g Fibre; 25 g Protein; 460 mg Sodium

Pictured on page 71 and on back cover.

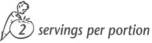

Thai Green Curry Beef

This rich and creamy coconut curry makes the perfect dinner companion for steamed white rice.

Cooking oil	1 tbsp.	15 mL
Ginger root slices, about 1/8 inch (3 mm) slices	4	4
Lemon grass, bulb only, quartered lengthwise	1	1
Thai hot chili pepper, finely chopped (see Tip, page 47)	1	1
Beef top sirloin steak, cut into thin strips	3/4 lb.	340 g
Can of coconut milk	14 oz.	398 mL
Can of cut baby corn, drained	14 oz.	398 mL
Chopped red pepper	1 cup	250 mL
Frozen peas, thawed	1 cup	250 mL
Can of shoestring-style bamboo shoots, drained	8 oz.	227 mL
Thai green curry paste	4 tsp.	20 mL
Brown sugar, packed	1 tbsp.	15 mL
Soy sauce	1 tbsp.	15 mL
Grated lime zest (see Tip, page 97)	1/2 tsp.	2 mL
Lime juice	1 tbsp.	15 mL
Finely shredded basil	2 tbsp.	30 mL

Heat cooking oil in large frying pan on medium-high. Add next 3 ingredients. Heat and stir for about 2 minutes until fragrant.

Add beef. Cook for about 3 minutes, stirring occasionally, until beef starts to brown. Reduce heat to medium.

Add next 9 ingredients. Stir. Cook for about 5 minutes, stirring occasionally, until red pepper is tender-crisp. Remove from heat. Remove and discard lemon grass and ginger root.

Add lime juice. Stir. Sprinkle with basil. Makes about 6 cups (1.5 L). Serves 4.

1 serving: 510 Calories; 34 g Total Fat (6 g Mono, 1.5 g Poly, 22 g Sat); 40 mg Cholesterol; 21 g Carbohydrate; 6 g Fibre; 24 g Protein; 780 mg Sodium

Pictured on page 71 and on back cover.

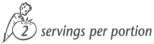

Steak and Radish Skewers

These attractive sesame-sprinkled skewers are packed with colourful vegetables and tender beef. Grilling radishes brings out their sweetness while retaining that peppery bite.

Asian-style sesame dressing	1 cup	250 mL
Soy sauce	1 tbsp.	15 mL
Rice vinegar	1 tsp.	5 mL
Ground ginger	1/2 tsp.	2 mL
Garlic powder	1/8 tsp.	0.5 mL
Beef strip loin steak, cut into 16 equal pieces	1 lb.	454 g
Large radishes, halved	16	16
Small whole fresh white mushrooms	16	16
Large green pepper, cut into 16 equal pieces	1	1
Bamboo skewers (8 inches, 20 cm, each), soaked in water for 10 minutes	8	8
Roasted sesame seeds	2 tsp.	10 mL

Combine first 5 ingredients in medium bowl. Reserve 1/3 cup (75 mL) in small cup.

Add beef to remaining dressing mixture. Stir. Marinate, covered, in refrigerator for 30 minutes, stirring once. Remove beef. Discard any remaining marinade.

Thread next 3 ingredients and beef alternately onto skewers. Preheat gas barbecue to medium-high. Place skewers on greased grill. Close lid. Cook for about 12 minutes, turning often, for medium or until beef reaches desired doneness and vegetables are tender-crisp. Brush with reserved dressing mixture.

Sprinkle with sesame seeds. Makes 8 skewers. Serves 4.

1 serving: 330 Calories; 11 g Total Fat (4.5 g Mono, 1 g Poly, 4 g Sat); 70 mg Cholesterol; 18 g Carbohydrate; 2 g Fibre; 36 g Protein; 580 mg Sodium

Pictured on page 71 and on back cover.

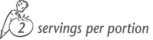
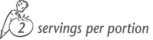 *servings per portion*

Below-ground Stew

This classic root stew contains all the best veggies grown below ground, and is guaranteed to satisfy the whole family—the kids will eat their veggies without argument!

All-purpose flour	1/4 cup	60 mL
Montreal steak spice	1/2 tsp.	2 mL
Stewing beef, trimmed of fat	1 1/2 lbs.	680 g
Chopped peeled potato	2 cups	500 mL
Sliced carrot	2 cups	500 mL
Chopped celery root	1 cup	250 mL
Chopped onion	1 cup	250 mL
Chopped yellow turnip (rutabaga)	1 cup	250 mL
Prepared beef broth	2 cups	500 mL
Tomato paste (see Tip, page 32)	2 tbsp.	30 mL
Ketchup	1 tbsp.	15 mL

Combine flour and steak spice in large resealable freezer bag. Add beef. Seal bag. Toss until coated. Transfer beef to greased 4 quart (4 L) casserole. Reserve remaining flour mixture.

Scatter next 5 ingredients over beef.

Whisk remaining 3 ingredients and reserved flour mixture in small bowl until smooth. Pour over vegetables. Cook, covered, in 350°F (175°C) oven for about 2 1/2 hours until beef is tender. Stir. Makes about 6 cups (1.5 L). Serves 6.

1 serving: 270 Calories; 8 g Total Fat (3 g Mono, 0 g Poly, 3 g Sat); 55 mg Cholesterol; 20 g Carbohydrate; 3 g Fibre; 28 g Protein; 450 mg Sodium

Pictured on page 35.

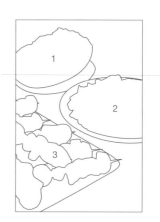

1. Stuffed Tuscan Squash, page 67
2. Thai Green Curry Beef, page 68
3. Steak and Radish Skewers, page 69

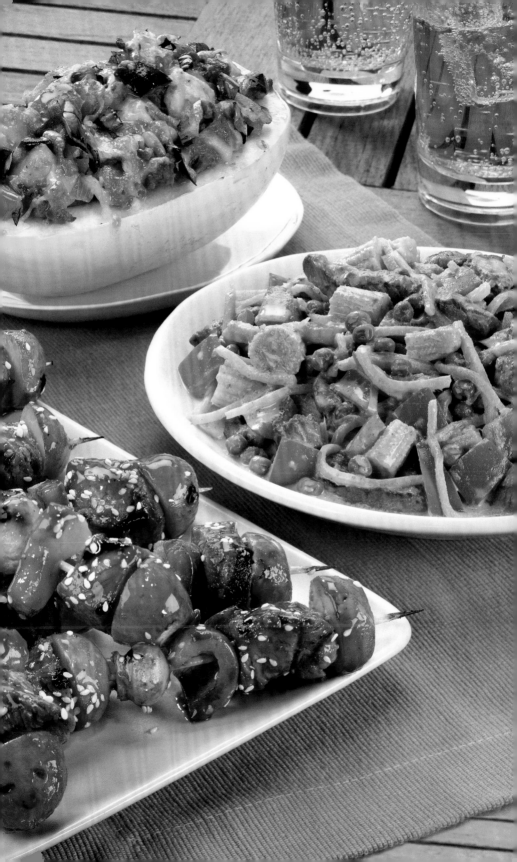

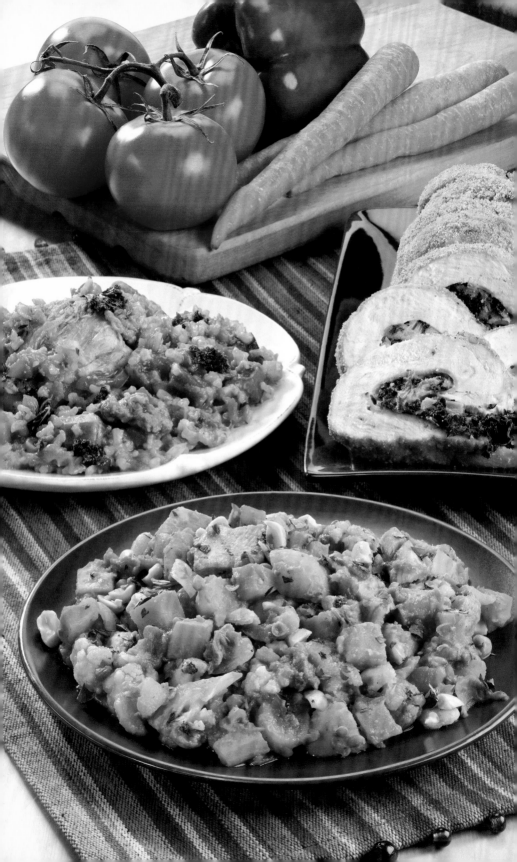

Chicken Veggie Meatballs

Meatballs are always a favourite with the kids, but these lean morsels have an edge up on the competition: they've got the added flavour and nutritional benefit of fresh veggies.

Large egg, fork-beaten	1	1
Fine dry bread crumbs	1/2 cup	125 mL
Grated carrot	1/2 cup	125 mL
Grated zucchini (with peel)	1/2 cup	125 mL
Grated Parmesan cheese	2 tbsp.	30 mL
Italian seasoning	1 tsp.	5 mL
Salt	1/4 tsp.	1 mL
Lean ground chicken	1 lb.	454 g
Tomato pasta sauce	2 3/4 cups	675 mL

Combine first 7 ingredients in large bowl.

Add chicken. Mix well. Roll into 1 inch (2.5 cm) balls. Arrange in single layer on greased baking sheet with sides. Broil on top rack in oven for about 7 minutes until no longer pink inside. Makes about 56 meatballs.

Bring sauce to a boil in medium saucepan. Add meatballs. Stir. Makes about 6 cups (1.5 L). Serves 6.

1 serving: 250 Calories; 6 g Total Fat (0.5 g Mono, 0 g Poly, 2 g Sat); 80 mg Cholesterol; 26 g Carbohydrate; 4 g Fibre; 22 g Protein; 750 mg Sodium

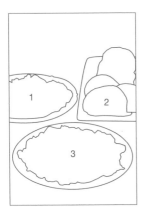

1. Creole Chicken Jambalaya, page 74
2. Cordon Spinach Turkey Roll, page 76
3. Nutty Turkey Stew, page 77

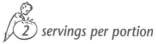

Creole Chicken Jambalaya

Everyone loves the spicy flavours of jambalaya, and you'll appreciate that this full-meal recipe features healthy doses of okra, tomatoes, celery, green pepper and onion.

Cooking oil	1 tbsp.	15 mL
Bone-in chicken thighs (about 5 – 6 oz., 140 – 170 g, each), skin removed	6	6
Chopped celery	1 cup	250 mL
Chopped green pepper	1 cup	250 mL
Chopped onion	1 cup	250 mL
Hot Italian sausage, casing removed	1/2 lb.	225 g
Can of diced tomatoes (with juice)	28 oz.	796 mL
Sliced fresh (or frozen) okra	2 cups	500 mL
Prepared chicken broth	1 1/4 cups	300 mL
Chopped kale leaves, lightly packed (see Tip, page 131)	1 cup	250 mL
Tomato paste (see Tip, page 32)	3 tbsp.	45 mL
Dried thyme	1 tsp.	5 mL
Hot pepper sauce	1 tsp.	5 mL
Worcestershire sauce	1 tsp.	5 mL
Garlic cloves, minced (or 1/2 tsp., 2 mL, powder)	2	2
Granulated sugar	1/2 tsp.	2 mL
Long-grain white rice	3/4 cup	175 mL
Bay leaf	1	1

Heat cooking oil in Dutch oven on medium-high. Add chicken. Cook for about 8 minutes, turning occasionally, until browned. Transfer to large plate. Reduce heat to medium.

Add next 4 ingredients to same pot. Scramble-fry for about 8 minutes until sausage is no longer pink.

Add next 10 ingredients. Heat and stir, scraping any brown bits from bottom of pan, until boiling.

(continued on next page)

Add rice, bay leaf and chicken. Stir. Bring to a boil. Reduce heat to medium-low. Simmer, covered, without stirring, for about 30 minutes until rice is tender and internal temperature of chicken reaches 170°F (77°C). Remove and discard bay leaf. Makes about 10 cups (2.5 L). Serves 6.

1 serving: 470 Calories; 19 g Total Fat (3.5 g Mono, 2 g Poly, 6 g Sat); 145 mg Cholesterol; 35 g Carbohydrate; 4 g Fibre; 39 g Protein; 1260 mg Sodium

Pictured on page 72.

Artichoke-stuffed Chicken

Stuff half a serving of vegetables into each tender chicken breast—now that's a clever method for sneaking extra veggies into your diet!

Egg yolk (large), fork-beaten	1	1
Jar of marinated artichoke hearts, drained and chopped	6 oz.	170 mL
Chopped arugula, lightly packed	1/2 cup	125 mL
Ricotta cheese	1/4 cup	60 mL
Sliced green olives, chopped	2 tbsp.	30 mL
Garlic clove, minced (or 1/4 tsp., 1 mL, powder)	1	1
Salt	1/8 tsp.	0.5 mL
Pepper	1/4 tsp.	1 mL
Boneless, skinless chicken breast halves (4 – 6 oz., 113 – 170 g, each)	4	4
Grated Parmesan cheese	2 tbsp.	30 mL

Combine first 8 ingredients in medium bowl.

Cut horizontal slits in thickest part of chicken breasts to create pockets. Fill with artichoke mixture. Secure with wooden picks. Preheat gas barbecue to medium. Place chicken on greased grill. Close lid. Cook for about 8 minutes per side until internal temperature of chicken (not stuffing) reaches 170°F (77°C).

Sprinkle with Parmesan cheese. Serves 4.

1 serving: 190 Calories; 6 g Total Fat (2 g Mono, 0.5 g Poly, 2 g Sat); 125 mg Cholesterol; 3 g Carbohydrate; 1 g Fibre; 30 g Protein; 400 mg Sodium

Cordon Spinach Turkey Roll

Presentation is everything, and these divine spiral slices are perfect for serving to company. Plus, they're delicious.

Cooking oil	2 tsp.	10 mL
Chopped onion	1 cup	250 mL
Grated carrot	1/3 cup	75 mL
Finely chopped celery	1/4 cup	60 mL
Box of frozen chopped spinach, thawed and squeezed dry	10 oz.	300 g
Crushed seasoned croutons	1/4 cup	60 mL
Prepared chicken broth	2 tbsp.	30 mL
Boneless, skinless turkey breast roast	2 lbs.	900 g
Deli ham slices (about 5 oz., 140 g)	4	4
Deli Swiss cheese slices (about 4 oz., 113 g)	5	5
Large egg, fork-beaten	1	1
Crushed seasoned croutons	1 cup	250 mL

Heat cooking oil in large frying pan on medium. Add next 3 ingredients. Cook for about 8 minutes, stirring often, until softened.

Add next 3 ingredients. Stir. Cool.

To butterfly turkey, cut horizontally lengthwise almost, but not quite through, to other side. Open flat. Place between 2 sheets of plastic wrap. Pound with mallet or rolling pin to 1/2 inch (12 mm) thickness. Arrange ham and cheese slices over cut side of turkey. Spread spinach mixture over cheese. Roll up tightly, jelly-roll style, starting from long edge. Tie with butcher's string at 1 inch (2.5 cm) intervals.

Brush turkey roll with egg. Discard any remaining egg.

Spread croutons on large sheet of waxed paper. Press turkey roll into croutons until coated. Discard any remaining croutons. Place turkey roll, seam-side down, on greased wire rack set in large roasting pan. Cook, uncovered, in 350°F (175°C) oven for about 85 minutes until internal temperature of turkey (not stuffing) reaches 170°F (77°C). Transfer to cutting board. Cover with foil. Let stand for 10 minutes. Remove and discard string. Cut into 3/4 inch (2 cm) slices. Serves 8.

(continued on next page)

1 serving: 320 Calories; 15 g Total Fat (6 g Mono, 2.5 g Poly, 5 g Sat); 110 mg Cholesterol; 9 g Carbohydrate; 2 g Fibre; 34 g Protein; 560 mg Sodium

Pictured on page 72.

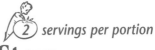 *servings per portion*

Nutty Turkey Stew

This flavourful offering puts all that leftover holiday turkey to good use—and it's healthy too! Serve over couscous to make a complete meal.

Cooking oil	1 tsp.	5 mL
Chopped carrot	1 cup	250 mL
Chopped onion	1 cup	250 mL
Ground cumin	2 tsp.	10 mL
Garlic cloves, minced	2	2
(or 1/2 tsp., 2 mL, powder)		
Ground cinnamon	1/4 tsp.	1 mL
Salt	1/2 tsp.	2 mL
Pepper	1/8 tsp.	0.5 mL
Can of diced tomatoes (with juice)	28 oz.	796 mL
Can of lentils, rinsed and drained	19 oz.	540 mL
Chopped cooked turkey (see Tip, page 101)	2 cups	500 mL
Small cauliflower florets	2 cups	500 mL
Chopped dried apricot	1/2 cup	125 mL
Peanut butter	1/4 cup	60 mL
Coarsely chopped unsalted peanuts	1/4 cup	60 mL
Chopped fresh parsley	2 tbsp.	30 mL

Heat cooking oil in Dutch oven on medium. Add next 7 ingredients. Cook for about 8 minutes, stirring often, until onion is softened.

Add next 6 ingredients. Stir. Bring to a boil. Reduce heat to medium-low. Simmer, covered, for about 30 minutes until cauliflower and carrot are tender-crisp.

Scatter peanuts and parsley over top. Makes about 7 1/2 cups (1.9 L). Serves 6.

1 serving: 280 Calories; 11 g Total Fat (2.5 g Mono, 1.5 g Poly, 2 g Sat); 20 mg Cholesterol; 30 g Carbohydrate; 10 g Fibre; 20 g Protein; 770 mg Sodium

Pictured on page 72.

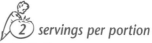
Turkey Veggie Cobbler

*Hate cooking a whole turkey because you never know what to do with all the
leftovers? Put them to good use in this delightful, veggie-packed offering that's
sure to appeal to the entire family.*

Cooking oil	2 tsp.	10 mL
Sliced leek (white part only)	2 cups	500 mL
Diced celery root	1 cup	250 mL
Salt	1/4 tsp.	1 mL
Pepper	1/4 tsp.	1 mL
Chopped cooked turkey (see Tip, page 101)	2 cups	500 mL
Frozen peas	2 cups	500 mL
Chopped seeded tomato	1 cup	250 mL
Prepared chicken broth	1/3 cup	75 mL
All-purpose flour	1 cup	250 mL
Baking powder	2 tsp.	10 mL
Dried oregano	1/2 tsp.	2 mL
Dried thyme	1/2 tsp.	2 mL
Salt	1/4 tsp.	1 mL
Cold butter (or hard margarine), cut up	1/3 cup	75 mL
Large egg, fork-beaten	1	1
Milk	2/3 cup	150 mL

Heat cooking oil in large frying pan on medium. Add next 4 ingredients.
Cook for about 10 minutes, stirring occasionally, until celery root starts to
soften.

Add next 4 ingredients. Cook for about 5 minutes, stirring occasionally,
until celery root is softened. Transfer to ungreased 2 quart (2 L) casserole.

Combine next 5 ingredients in medium bowl. Cut in butter until mixture
resembles coarse crumbs. Make a well in centre.

Add egg and milk to well. Stir until just moistened. Drop by mounded
spoonfuls over hot turkey mixture. Bake, uncovered, in 400°F (200°C) oven
for about 25 minutes until golden and wooden pick inserted in centre of
biscuit comes out clean. Serves 6.

*1 serving: 300 Calories; 14 g Total Fat (4 g Mono, 1 g Poly, 7 g Sat); 75 mg Cholesterol;
28 g Carbohydrate; 4 g Fibre; 16 g Protein; 530 mg Sodium*

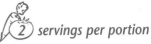

Chicken and Eggplant Curry

If it's curry you crave, it's curry you'll get! Serve this saucy dish with steamed rice for a fab meal.

Cooking oil	2 tsp.	10 mL
Sliced Asian eggplant (with peel), about 1/2 inch (12 mm) slices	4 cups	1 L
Sliced onion	1 1/2 cups	375 mL
Mild curry paste	2 tbsp.	30 mL
Finely grated ginger root (or 1/2 tsp., 2 mL, ground ginger)	2 tsp.	10 mL
Garlic clove, minced (or 1/4 tsp., 1 mL, powder)	1	1
Ground cumin	1 tsp.	5 mL
Ground cinnamon	1/2 tsp.	2 mL
Salt	1/8 tsp.	0.5 mL
Boneless, skinless chicken thighs, quartered	1 1/2 lbs.	680 g
Coconut milk	1 cup	250 mL
Prepared chicken broth	2/3 cup	150 mL
Brown sugar, packed	1 tbsp.	15 mL
Chopped tomato	1 cup	250 mL
Frozen cut green beans, thawed	1 cup	250 mL
Chopped salted cashews	2 tbsp.	30 mL
Chopped fresh cilantro (or parsley)	1 tbsp.	15 mL

Heat cooking oil in large saucepan on medium. Add eggplant and onion. Cook for about 15 minutes, stirring often, until softened and starting to brown.

Add next 6 ingredients. Heat and stir for about 2 minutes until fragrant.

Add next 4 ingredients. Stir. Cook, covered, for about 15 minutes, stirring occasionally, until chicken is no longer pink inside.

Add tomato and green beans. Stir. Cook, covered, for about 5 minutes, stirring occasionally, until green beans are tender-crisp.

Sprinkle with cashews and cilantro. Makes about 6 cups (1.5 L). Serves 6.

1 serving: 310 Calories; 17 g Total Fat (3.5 g Mono, 2 g Poly, 9 g Sat); 95 mg Cholesterol; 15 g Carbohydrate; 5 g Fibre; 25 g Protein; 530 mg Sodium

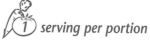
Swiss Chard Chicken Rolls

Filled with a delicious mixture of chicken, bacon and rice, these rolls are similar to cabbage rolls—though surrounded with leaves of Swiss chard instead!

Water	1 cup	250 mL
Diced onion	1 cup	250 mL
Short-grain white rice	1 cup	250 mL
Diced celery	1/2 cup	125 mL
Lean ground chicken	3/4 lb.	340 g
Bacon slices, cooked crisp and crumbled	3	3
Salt	1/2 tsp.	2 mL
Pepper	1/2 tsp.	2 mL
Garlic clove, minced (or 1/4 tsp., 1 mL, powder)	1	1
Large Swiss chard leaves, ribs removed (see Tip, page 131)	12	12
Water	1 tbsp.	15 mL
Prepared chicken broth	1/2 cup	125 mL
Sour cream	3/4 cup	175 mL
Lemon wedges	6	6

Bring water to a boil in medium saucepan. Add next 3 ingredients. Stir. Reduce heat to medium-low. Simmer, covered, for 10 minutes, without stirring. Remove from heat. Let stand, covered, for about 5 minutes until liquid is absorbed. Rice will be partially cooked. Transfer to large bowl. Cool completely.

Add next 5 ingredients. Mix well.

Stack chard leaves in large microwave-safe bowl. Sprinkle with water. Microwave, covered, on high (100%) for about 3 minutes until leaves are wilted (see Tip, page 119). Let stand until cool enough to handle. Drain. Place about 1/3 cup (75 mL) rice mixture on 1 chard leaf. Fold in sides. Roll up tightly from bottom to enclose. Repeat with remaining rice mixture and chard leaves. Arrange rolls, seam-side down, in single layer in greased 3 quart (3 L) casserole.

Pour broth over top. Cook, covered, in 350°F (175°C) oven for about 1 hour until internal temperature reaches 175°F (80°C).

(continued on next page)

Serve with sour cream and lemon wedges. Makes 12 rolls. Serves 6.

1 serving: 300 Calories; 9 g Total Fat (2.5 g Mono, 0.5 g Poly, 4.5 g Sat); 55 mg Cholesterol; 36 g Carbohydrate; 3 g Fibre; 19 g Protein; 590 mg Sodium

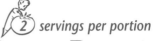 *servings per portion*

Citrus Chicken and Green Beans

Deliciously fresh citrus flavours work their magic on tender chicken and crisp green beans. Serve this delightful dish over rice.

Cooking oil	1 tbsp.	15 mL
Boneless, skinless chicken thighs, quartered	1 lb.	454 g
Chopped onion	1 cup	250 mL
Garlic cloves, minced	2	2
(or 1/2 tsp., 2 mL, powder)		
All-purpose flour	1 tbsp.	15 mL
Pepper	1/4 tsp.	1 mL
Prepared chicken broth	1 cup	250 mL
Frozen concentrated orange juice, thawed	2 tbsp.	30 mL
Fresh (or frozen) whole green beans, halved	3 cups	750 mL
Grated lemon zest	1 tsp.	5 mL
Grated orange zest	1 tsp.	5 mL

Heat cooking oil in large frying pan on medium-high. Add chicken. Cook for about 5 minutes, stirring occasionally, until browned. Transfer to small bowl. Cover to keep warm. Reduce heat to medium.

Add onion and garlic to same frying pan. Cook for about 3 minutes, stirring often, until onion is softened.

Add flour and pepper. Heat and stir for 1 minute. Slowly add broth and concentrated orange juice, stirring constantly until smooth. Heat and stir until boiling and thickened.

Add green beans and chicken. Stir. Boil gently, covered, for about 6 minutes until chicken is no longer pink inside and green beans are tender-crisp.

Add lemon zest and orange zest. Stir. Makes about 4 cups (1 L). Serves 4.

1 serving: 230 Calories; 8 g Total Fat (3.5 g Mono, 2 g Poly, 1.5 g Sat); 95 mg Cholesterol; 14 g Carbohydrate; 3 g Fibre; 25 g Protein; 480 mg Sodium

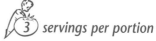

Snap Pea Chicken Skillet

Tender chicken in a flavourful sauce of wine and dill makes the perfect dinner companion for rice.

All-purpose flour	2 tbsp.	30 mL
Salt	1/2 tsp.	2 mL
Pepper	1/2 tsp.	2 mL
Boneless, skinless chicken breast halves, cut crosswise into 1/2 inch (12 mm) slices	1 lb.	454 g
Cooking oil	1 tbsp.	15 mL
Cooking oil	2 tsp.	10 mL
Sliced fresh white mushrooms	3 cups	750 mL
Chopped onion	1 cup	250 mL
Dry (or alcohol-free) white wine	1/3 cup	75 mL
Prepared chicken broth	1/3 cup	75 mL
Butter (or hard margarine)	1 tbsp.	15 mL
Lemon juice	1 tbsp.	15 mL
Grated lemon zest (see Tip, page 97)	1 tsp.	5 mL
Sugar snap peas, trimmed	3 cups	750 mL
Chopped fresh dill (or 3/4 tsp., 4 mL, dried)	1 tbsp.	15 mL
Salt	1/2 tsp.	2 mL
Pepper	1/4 tsp.	1 mL

Combine first 3 ingredients in large resealable freezer bag. Add chicken. Toss until coated. Remove chicken. Discard any remaining flour mixture.

Heat cooking oil in large frying pan on medium-high. Add chicken. Cook for about 5 minutes, stirring occasionally, until browned. Transfer to small bowl. Cover to keep warm. Reduce heat to medium.

Add second amount of cooking oil to same frying pan. Add mushrooms and onion. Cook for about 3 minutes, stirring occasionally, until mushrooms start to brown.

Add next 5 ingredients. Stir. Bring to a boil.

Add remaining 4 ingredients and chicken. Heat and stir for about 3 minutes until chicken is no longer pink inside and peas are tender-crisp. Makes about 6 1/2 cups (1.6 L). Serves 4.

(continued on next page)

1 serving: 330 Calories; 10 g Total Fat (4.5 g Mono, 2 g Poly, 2.5 g Sat); 75 mg Cholesterol; 20 g Carbohydrate; 3 g Fibre; 31 g Protein; 800 mg Sodium

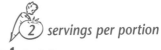 *2 servings per portion*

Turkey Cacciatore

Serve this saucy favourite over pasta or rice.

Cooking oil	2 tsp.	10 mL
Boneless, skinless turkey thighs, cut into 1 1/2 inch (3.8 cm) pieces	1 1/2 lbs.	680 g
Salt	1/2 tsp.	2 mL
Pepper	1/4 tsp.	1 mL
Halved fresh white mushrooms	2 cups	500 mL
Chopped onion	1 cup	250 mL
Sliced celery	1/2 cup	125 mL
Garlic clove, minced (or 1/4 tsp., 1 mL, powder)	1	1
Dry (or alcohol-free) white wine	1/2 cup	125 mL
Can of diced tomatoes (with juice)	28 oz.	796 mL
Diced yellow pepper	1 1/2 cups	375 mL
Tomato paste (see Tip, page 32)	1/4 cup	60 mL
Dried basil	1 tsp.	5 mL
Granulated sugar	1 tsp.	5 mL
Grated Parmesan cheese	1/4 cup	60 mL

Heat cooking oil in Dutch oven on medium-high. Add turkey. Sprinkle with salt and pepper. Cook for about 5 minutes, stirring occasionally, until starting to brown. Reduce heat to medium.

Add next 4 ingredients. Cook for about 10 minutes, stirring occasionally, until onion is softened and liquid has evaporated.

Add wine. Heat and stir for 1 minute. Add next 5 ingredients. Stir. Bring to a boil. Reduce heat to medium-low. Simmer, partially covered, for about 45 minutes, stirring occasionally, until turkey is tender.

Add cheese. Stir. Makes about 7 cups (1.75 L). Serves 6.

1 serving: 250 Calories; 8 g Total Fat (3.5 g Mono, 1.5 g Poly, 2 g Sat); 95 mg Cholesterol; 15 g Carbohydrate; 3 g Fibre; 26 g Protein; 740 mg Sodium

Pictured on page 126.

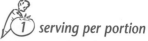

Salmon with Cucumber Salsa

Simple broiled salmon is elevated to company quality with the addition of a summery salsa of sweet corn, crisp cucumber, red pepper and onion.

Finely chopped seeded English cucumber (with peel)	1 1/2 cups	375 mL
Fresh (or frozen, thawed) kernel corn	1/2 cup	125 mL
Finely chopped red pepper	1/3 cup	75 mL
Finely chopped red onion	1/4 cup	60 mL
Mayonnaise	2 tbsp.	30 mL
Chopped fresh parsley (or 3/4 tsp., 4 mL, flakes)	1 tbsp.	15 mL
Sweet chili sauce	1 tbsp.	15 mL
White wine vinegar	2 tsp.	10 mL
Chopped fresh basil (or 1/4 tsp., 1 mL, dried)	1 tsp.	5 mL
Salt	1/8 tsp.	0.5 mL
Salmon fillets (4 – 5 oz., 113 – 140 g, each), any small bones removed	4	4
Salt, sprinkle		
Pepper, sprinkle		

Combine first 10 ingredients in small bowl. Makes about 2 cups (500 mL) salsa.

Sprinkle fillets with salt and pepper. Arrange on greased baking sheet with sides. Broil on top rack in oven for about 5 minutes until fish flakes easily when tested with fork. Serve with salsa. Serves 4.

1 serving: 250 Calories; 13 g Total Fat (2.5 g Mono, 3 g Poly, 2 g Sat); 65 mg Cholesterol; 9 g Carbohydrate; 1 g Fibre; 24 g Protein; 180 mg Sodium

Pictured on page 89.

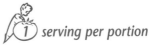

Corn-crusted Tilapia

Cornmeal provides a crispy crust for this kid-friendly dish of baked fish and tender veggies. More than one serving of vegetables hides with each serving of fish.

Cooking oil	1 tsp.	5 mL
Chopped onion	1/2 cup	125 mL
Chopped fresh (or frozen, thawed) whole green beans	1 cup	250 mL
Fresh (or frozen, thawed) kernel corn	1 cup	250 mL
Chopped red pepper	1/2 cup	125 mL
Italian dressing	2 tbsp.	30 mL
Large egg	1	1
Taco seasoning mix, stir before measuring	2 tbsp.	30 mL
Yellow cornmeal	2 tbsp.	30 mL
All-purpose flour	1 tbsp.	15 mL
Tilapia fillets, any small bones removed	1 lb.	454 g
Cooking oil	1 tbsp.	15 mL

Heat first amount of cooking oil in medium frying pan. Add onion. Cook for about 5 minutes, stirring often, until softened.

Add next 3 ingredients. Cook for about 5 minutes, stirring occasionally, until red pepper is tender-crisp.

Add dressing. Heat and stir for 1 minute. Remove from heat. Cover to keep warm. Makes about 2 1/4 cups (550 mL) vegetables.

Beat egg with fork in medium shallow dish.

Combine next 3 ingredients in separate medium shallow dish.

Dip fillets into egg. Press both sides into cornmeal mixture until coated. Discard any remaining cornmeal mixture.

Heat second amount of cooking oil in large frying pan on medium. Add fillets. Cook for about 3 minutes per side until golden and fish flakes easily when tested with fork. Serve fillets with vegetable mixture. Serves 4.

1 serving: 270 Calories; 9 g Total Fat (3.5 g Mono, 1.5 g Poly, 1 g Sat); 100 mg Cholesterol; 21 g Carbohydrate; 2 g Fibre; 25 g Protein; 460 mg Sodium

Pictured on page 89.

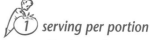

Coconut Curry Shrimp Stir-fry

*Stir things up with this sweet curry stir-fry. Packed with tender shrimp,
this dish makes for an inviting and fresh-looking meal option.
Serve over steamed rice.*

Can of coconut milk	14 oz.	398 mL
Cornstarch	1 tbsp.	15 mL
Curry powder	1 tbsp.	15 mL
Salt	1/2 tsp.	2 mL
Garlic powder	1/4 tsp.	1 mL
Cooking oil	1 tbsp.	15 mL
Chopped cabbage	2 cups	500 mL
Broccoli florets	1 cup	250 mL
Chopped bok choy	1 cup	250 mL
Sliced onion	1/2 cup	125 mL
Sliced red pepper	1/2 cup	125 mL
Thinly sliced carrot, cut diagonally	1/2 cup	125 mL
Uncooked large shrimp (peeled and deveined)	1 lb.	454 g

Whisk first 5 ingredients in medium bowl.

Heat large frying pan or wok on medium-high until very hot. Add cooking
oil. Add next 6 ingredients. Stir-fry for 3 minutes. Stir cornstarch mixture.
Add to vegetable mixture. Stir-fry for about 1 minute until boiling
and thickened.

Add shrimp. Stir. Cook for about 3 minutes, stirring occasionally, until
shrimp turn pink. Makes about 7 cups (1.75 L). Serves 6.

*1 serving: 260 Calories; 18 g Total Fat (2 g Mono, 1.5 g Poly, 13 g Sat); 115 mg Cholesterol;
10 g Carbohydrate; 2 g Fibre; 18 g Protein; 300 mg Sodium*

Pictured on page 89.

 HELPFUL **H**INTS Bok choy is a soft but crunchy vegetable. Its name sounds quite
exotic, but actually means "white vegetable" in Cantonese.

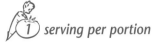
Shrimp and Artichoke Risotto

Rich and creamy risotto is always an elegant main course—perfect for serving company. Tender shrimp, tangy artichoke, and a lovely herb flavour make this recipe unforgettable.

Prepared vegetable broth	6 cups	1.5 L
Cooking oil	1 tbsp.	15 mL
Chopped onion	1 cup	250 mL
Arborio rice	1 1/2 cups	375 mL
Grated zucchini (with peel)	1 cup	250 mL
Garlic clove, minced	1	1
(or 1/4 tsp., 1 mL, powder)		
Coarsely ground pepper	1/4 tsp.	1 mL
Cooked medium shrimp	1 lb.	454 g
(peeled and deveined)		
Can of artichoke hearts, drained	14 oz.	398 mL
and quartered		
Halved grape tomatoes	1 cup	250 mL
Goat (chèvre) cheese, cut up	2 oz.	57 g
Chopped fresh parsley	3 tbsp.	45 mL
White wine vinegar	1 tbsp.	15 mL

Bring broth to a boil in medium saucepan. Reduce heat to low. Cover to keep hot.

Heat cooking oil in large saucepan on medium. Add onion. Cook for about 5 minutes, stirring often, until onion is softened.

Add next 4 ingredients. Heat and stir for about 1 minute until rice is coated and garlic is fragrant. Add 1 cup (250 mL) of hot broth, stirring constantly until broth is absorbed. Repeat with remaining broth, 1 cup (250 mL) at a time, until broth is absorbed and rice is tender and creamy.

Add shrimp and artichoke hearts. Stir. Cook for about 3 minutes, stirring constantly, until heated through.

Add remaining 4 ingredients. Stir gently. Makes about 9 2/3 cups (2.4 L). Serves 6.

1 serving: 350 Calories; 6 g Total Fat (2 g Mono, 1 g Poly, 2 g Sat); 120 mg Cholesterol; 50 g Carbohydrate; 3 g Fibre; 22 g Protein; 850 mg Sodium

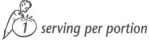

Jicama Salmon Cakes

Fishcakes with a facelift—these tasty salmon patties get their great texture from jicama. Zucchini pumps up the veggie factor even more, with dill and feta cheese rounding out the flavours.

Grated peeled jicama, squeezed dry	1 cup	250 mL
Grated zucchini (with peel), squeezed dry	1/2 cup	125 mL
Large egg, fork-beaten	1	1
Can of red salmon, drained, skin and round bones removed	7 1/2 oz.	213 g
Fine dry bread crumbs	1/2 cup	125 mL
Crumbled feta cheese	1/4 cup	60 mL
Dried dillweed	1/2 tsp.	2 mL
Garlic powder	1/8 tsp.	0.5 mL
Salt	1/4 tsp.	1 mL
Pepper	1/8 tsp.	0.5 mL
Cooking oil	1 tbsp.	15 mL

Lemon wedges, for garnish

Combine jicama and zucchini in large bowl.

Add next 8 ingredients. Mix well. Divide into 4 equal portions. Shape into 3 inch (7.5 cm) patties.

Heat cooking oil in large frying pan on medium. Add patties. Cook for about 5 minutes per side until browned. Makes 4 cakes. Serves 4.

1 serving: 190 Calories; 10 g Total Fat (3 g Mono, 1.5 g Poly, 3 g Sat); 60 mg Cholesterol; 15 g Carbohydrate; 3 g Fibre; 11 g Protein; 460 mg Sodium

1. Coconut Curry Shrimp Stir-fry, page 86
2. Corn-crusted Tilapia, page 85
3. Salmon with Cucumber Salsa, page 84

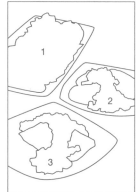

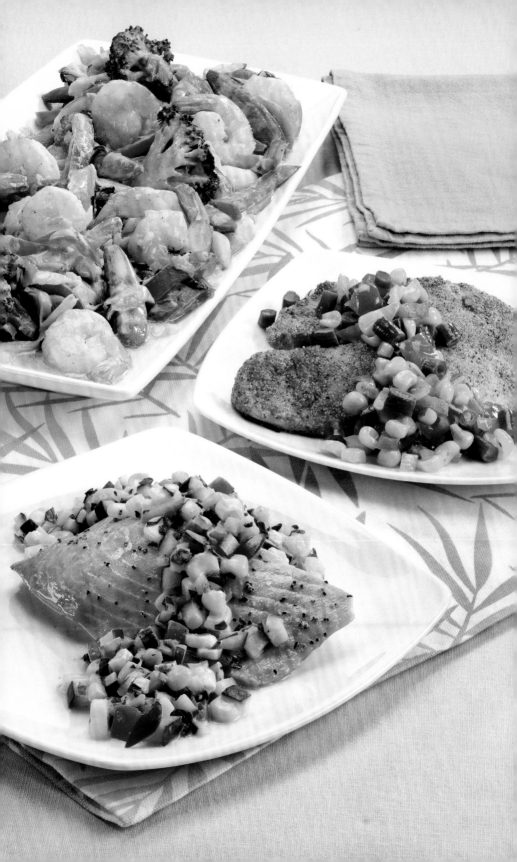

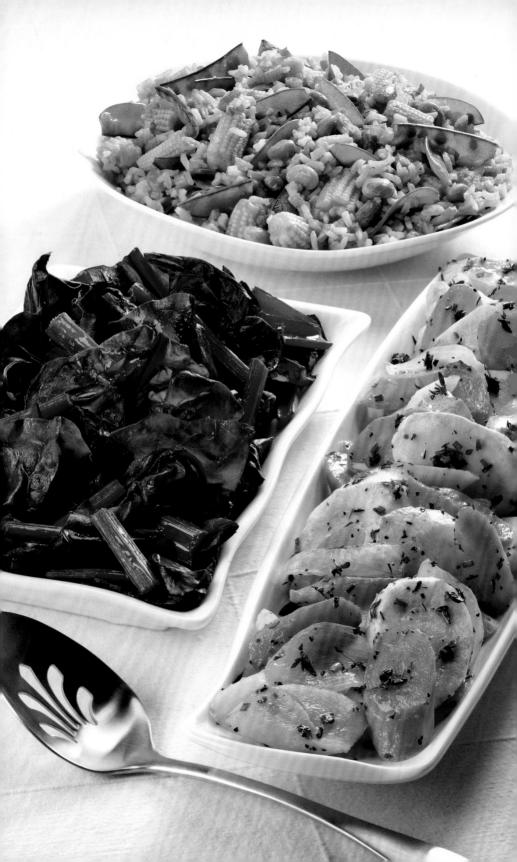

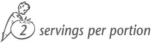

Snappy Scallop Stir-fry

A hearty dose of snap peas, mild bay scallops and a nice chili heat make for a memorable mixture that's best served over rice.

Prepared vegetable broth	1/3 cup	75 mL
Cornstarch	2 tsp.	10 mL
Finely grated ginger root	2 tsp.	10 mL
(or 1/2 tsp., 2 mL, ground ginger)		
Soy sauce	2 tsp.	10 mL
Garlic cloves, minced	2	2
(or 1/2 tsp., 2 mL, powder)		
Chili paste (sambal oelek)	1/2 tsp.	2 mL
Cooking oil	2 tsp.	10 mL
Sugar snap peas, trimmed	3 cups	750 mL
Chopped green onion (2 inch, 5 cm, pieces)	1/2 cup	125 mL
Julienned carrot (see Tip, page 15)	1/2 cup	125 mL
Small bay scallops	3/4 lb.	340 g

Combine first 6 ingredients in small bowl.

Heat large frying pan or wok on medium-high until very hot. Add cooking oil. Add next 3 ingredients. Stir-fry for about 3 minutes until peas are tender-crisp.

Add scallops. Stir-fry for 1 minute. Stir cornstarch mixture. Add to scallop mixture. Stir-fry for about 1 minute until scallops are opaque and sauce is boiling and thickened. Makes about 4 cups (1 L). Serves 4.

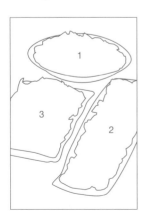

1 serving: 140 Calories; 3 g Total Fat (1.5 g Mono, 1 g Poly, 0 g Sat); 30 mg Cholesterol; 14 g Carbohydrate; 2 g Fibre; 17 g Protein; 490 mg Sodium

1. Veggie Fried Rice, page 132
2. Fragrant Herbed Vegetables, page 133
3. Raspberry Ruby Chard, page 131

Tuna Melt Calzone

Getting all your daily servings of veggies doesn't need to be difficult. This fun recipe has all the classic flavours of a tuna melt, and each slice sneaks in over half a serving of veggies. Kids will love the unique presentation.

All-purpose flour	2 cups	500 mL
Envelope of instant yeast	1/4 oz.	8 g
(or 2 1/4 tsp., 11 mL)		
Salt	1 tsp.	5 mL
Hot water (see Tip, page 51)	1/2 cup	125 mL
Mashed canned sweet potato	1/2 cup	125 mL
Cooking oil	2 tbsp.	30 mL
All-purpose flour, approximately	3 tbsp.	45 mL
Grated butternut squash (see Tip, page 33)	1 cup	250 mL
Grated medium Cheddar cheese	1 cup	250 mL
Can of chunk light tuna in water, drained	6 oz.	170 g
Chopped fresh white mushrooms	1/2 cup	125 mL
Basil pesto	2 tbsp.	30 mL
Thinly sliced green onion	2 tbsp.	30 mL
Large egg	1	1
Water	1 tbsp.	15 mL

Combine first 3 ingredients in large bowl. Make a well in centre.

Add hot water to well. Stir.

Add sweet potato and cooking oil. Mix until soft dough forms. Turn out onto lightly floured surface.

Knead for 5 to 10 minutes until smooth and elastic, adding second amount of all-purpose flour, 1 tbsp. (15 mL) at a time, if necessary, to prevent sticking. Place in greased large bowl, turning once to grease top. Cover with greased waxed paper and tea towel. Let stand in oven with light on and door closed for about 45 minutes until doubled in size. Punch dough down. Roll out to 14 inch (35 cm) circle. Carefully transfer to large greased baking sheet.

Combine next 6 ingredients in medium bowl. Spread over half of dough leaving 1 inch (2.5 cm) border.

(continued on next page)

Whisk egg and water in small bowl. Brush over edges of dough. Fold dough over filling. Press edges together with fork to seal. Brush remaining egg mixture over top. Cut 3 slits in top to allow steam to escape. Bake in 425°F (220°C) oven for about 20 minutes until bottom is golden. Let stand on pan for 10 minutes. Cuts into 6 slices. Serves 6.

1 serving: 380 Calories; 14 g Total Fat (4.5 g Mono, 2 g Poly, 4.5 g Sat); 50 mg Cholesterol; 45 g Carbohydrate; 3 g Fibre; 18 g Protein; 660 mg Sodium

 servings per portion

Braised Leek and Basa

Moist, perfectly cooked fish fillets rest on a bed of roasted leek and mushrooms. Subtle notes of lemon and tarragon contribute to this delicious and nutritious selection.

Thinly sliced leek (white part only)	3 cups	750 mL
Thinly sliced onion	1 cup	250 mL
Thinly sliced portobello mushrooms	1 cup	250 mL
Cooking oil	2 tbsp.	30 mL
Garlic clove, minced	1	1
(or 1/4 tsp., 1 mL, powder)		
Prepared chicken broth	1/2 cup	125 mL
Dry (or alcohol-free) white wine	1/4 cup	60 mL
Dried tarragon	1/2 tsp.	2 mL
Grated lemon zest	1/2 tsp.	2 mL
Basa fillets, any small bones removed	1 lb.	454 g
Salt	1/4 tsp.	1 mL
Pepper	1/8 tsp.	0.5 mL
Chopped fresh parsley	2 tbsp.	30 mL

Combine first 5 ingredients in large bowl. Transfer to ungreased 9 x 13 inch (23 x 33 cm) baking dish. Cook in 425°F (220°C) oven for about 25 minutes, stirring occasionally, until golden.

Add next 4 ingredients. Stir.

Arrange fillets over top. Sprinkle with salt and pepper. Cook for about 12 minutes until fish flakes easily when tested with fork.

Sprinkle with parsley. Makes about 2 cups (500 mL) vegetables. Serves 4.

1 serving: 270 Calories; 16 g Total Fat (8 g Mono, 3.5 g Poly, 2.5 g Sat); 55 mg Cholesterol; 9 g Carbohydrate; 2 g Fibre; 19 g Protein; 370 mg Sodium

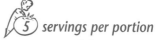

Baked Snapper Ratatouille

You can seriously increase your veggie intake with this smart and snappy ratatouille.

Chopped Asian eggplant (with peel)	3 cups	750 mL
Chopped zucchini (with peel)	3 cups	750 mL
Chopped red onion	1 cup	250 mL
Chopped red pepper	1 cup	250 mL
Olive (or cooking) oil	2 tbsp.	30 mL
Garlic cloves, chopped	2	2
(or 1/2 tsp., 2 mL, powder)		
Chopped tomato	2 cups	500 mL
Can of tomato sauce	7 1/2 oz.	213 mL
Dried dillweed	1 tsp.	5 mL
Grated lemon zest (see Tip, page 97)	1 tsp.	5 mL
Salt	1/2 tsp.	2 mL
Pepper	1/4 tsp.	1 mL
Chopped fresh basil	2 tbsp.	30 mL
Lemon juice	2 tbsp.	30 mL
Snapper fillets, any small bones removed	1 lb.	454 g
Salt, sprinkle		
Pepper, sprinkle		

Toss first 6 ingredients in large bowl. Transfer to ungreased 9 x 13 inch (23 x 33 cm) baking dish. Cook, uncovered, in 425°F (220°C) oven for about 25 minutes, stirring occasionally, until vegetables start to soften.

Add next 6 ingredients. Stir. Cook for 5 minutes.

Add basil and lemon juice. Stir.

Arrange fillets over top. Sprinkle with salt and pepper. Cook for about 5 minutes until fish flakes easily when tested with fork. Makes about 6 cups (1.5 L) eggplant mixture. Serves 4.

1 serving: 270 Calories; 9 g Total Fat (5 g Mono, 1.5 g Poly, 1.5 g Sat); 40 mg Cholesterol; 21 g Carbohydrate; 7 g Fibre; 28 g Protein; 610 mg Sodium

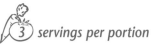

Cauliflower Fish Curry

Mild and tangy curry with lots of cauliflower and hearty bites of haddock.
This dish is light yet satisfying, and great served with rice or a spoonful of
plain yogurt.

Cooking oil	2 tsp.	10 mL
Chopped onion	1 cup	250 mL
Curry powder	1 tbsp.	15 mL
Ground cumin	1 tsp.	5 mL
Garlic powder	1/4 tsp.	1 mL
Salt	1/4 tsp.	1 mL
Pepper	1/4 tsp.	1 mL
All-purpose flour	1 tbsp.	15 mL
Cauliflower florets, halved	4 cups	1 L
Diced Roma (plum) tomato	1 1/2 cups	375 mL
Frozen pea and carrot mix	1 cup	250 mL
Prepared vegetable broth	1/2 cup	125 mL
Brown sugar, packed	4 tsp.	20 mL
Haddock fillets, any small bones removed, cut into 1 inch (2.5 cm) pieces	1 lb.	454 g
Chopped fresh cilantro (or parsley), optional	1 tbsp.	15 mL

Heat cooking oil in large saucepan on medium. Add next 6 ingredients. Cook for about 5 minutes, stirring often, until onion is softened.

Add flour. Heat and stir for 1 minute. Add next 5 ingredients. Stir. Bring to a boil on medium. Cook, covered, for about 8 minutes until cauliflower is tender-crisp.

Add fish. Stir. Cook, covered, for about 3 minutes until fish flakes easily when tested with fork.

Add cilantro. Stir. Makes about 6 cups (1.5 L). Serves 4.

1 serving: 230 Calories; 3.5 g Total Fat (1.5 g Mono, 1 g Poly, 0 g Sat); 65 mg Cholesterol; 24 g Carbohydrate; 5 g Fibre; 26 g Protein; 340 mg Sodium

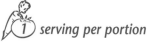
Lemon Lamb Shanks

This flavourful dish of melt-in-your-mouth lamb was inspired by the classic osso bucco, with a thick and fresh-tasting sauce of puréed carrot and onion.

Chopped fresh parsley	1/2 cup	125 mL
Grated lemon zest (see Tip, page 97)	1 tbsp.	15 mL
Lamb shanks (about 3 – 4 lbs., 1.4 – 1.8 kg), see Note	6	6
Salt	1/4 tsp.	1 mL
Pepper	1/4 tsp.	1 mL
Cooking oil	1 tsp.	5 mL
Chopped carrot	2 cups	500 mL
Sliced onion	2 cups	500 mL
Roasted garlic tomato pasta sauce	2 cups	500 mL
Dry (or alcohol-free) red wine	1 cup	250 mL
Water	1 cup	250 mL
Lemon juice	2 tbsp.	30 mL
Chopped fresh rosemary (or 3/4 tsp., 4 mL, dried, crushed)	1 tbsp.	15 mL
Boiling water	1 cup	250 mL

Combine parsley and lemon zest in small bowl. Chill, covered.

Sprinkle lamb with salt and pepper. Heat cooking oil in large frying pan on medium-high. Cook lamb in 2 batches, for about 8 minutes per batch, turning occasionally, until browned on all sides. Transfer to medium roasting pan. Drain and discard all but 1 tsp. (5 mL) drippings. Reduce heat to medium.

Add carrot and onion to same frying pan. Cook for about 12 minutes, stirring often, until onion is softened and starting to brown. Add to lamb.

Add next 5 ingredients to same frying pan. Heat and stir, scraping any brown bits from bottom of pan, until boiling. Pour over lamb. Cook, covered, in 350°F (175°C) oven for about 3 hours until lamb is tender. Transfer lamb to serving plate. Cover to keep warm. Skim and discard fat from cooking liquid.

(continued on next page)

Add boiling water to cooking liquid. Carefully process in blender in batches until smooth (see Safety Tip). Pour over lamb. Sprinkle with parsley mixture. Serves 6.

1 serving: 570 Calories; 23 g Total Fat (7 g Mono, 1 g Poly, 7 g Sat); 190 mg Cholesterol; 17 g Carbohydrate; 4 g Fibre; 64 g Protein; 570 mg Sodium

Note: Lamb shanks are commonly found in frozen bulk packages. If using frozen shanks, remember to thaw them before using.

Safety Tip: Follow manufacturer's instructions for processing hot liquids.

 When a recipe calls for grated zest and juice, it's easier to grate the fruit first, then juice it. Be careful not to grate down to the pith (white part of the peel), which is bitter and best avoided.

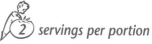

Curried Lamb and Fennel

Aromatic and attractive orange curry with green spinach and tender bites of lamb. Serve this super saucy dish over basmati rice to make a complete meal.

Cooking oil	2 tsp.	10 mL
Sliced fennel bulb (white part only)	3 cups	750 mL
Sliced onion	1 cup	250 mL
Mild curry paste	2 tbsp.	30 mL
All-purpose flour	1 tbsp.	15 mL
Garlic cloves, minced	2	2
(or 1/2 tsp., 2 mL, powder)		
Liquid honey	1 tsp.	5 mL
Whole green cardamom, bruised	1	1
(see Note)		
Dry mustard	1/2 tsp.	2 mL
Grated lemon zest	1/2 tsp.	2 mL
Salt	1/2 tsp.	2 mL
Pepper	1/2 tsp.	2 mL
Turmeric	1/2 tsp.	2 mL
Lamb shoulder, trimmed of fat and cut into 1 inch (2.5 cm) pieces	1 lb.	454 g
Water	1 cup	250 mL
Chopped fresh spinach leaves, lightly packed	2 cups	500 mL
Half-and-half cream	1/2 cup	125 mL

Heat cooking oil in large saucepan on medium. Add fennel and onion. Cook for about 10 minutes, stirring often, until fennel starts to soften.

Add next 10 ingredients. Heat and stir for about 1 minute until fragrant.

Add lamb and water. Stir. Cook, covered, for about 45 minutes until lamb is tender. Remove and discard cardamom. Remove from heat.

Add spinach and cream. Stir. Let stand, covered, for about 5 minutes until spinach is wilted. Makes about 5 cups (1.25 L). Serves 4.

1 serving: 280 Calories; 14 g Total Fat (4 g Mono, 1 g Poly, 4.5 g Sat); 90 mg Cholesterol; 13 g Carbohydrate; 4 g Fibre; 25 g Protein; 680 mg Sodium

Note: To bruise cardamom, pound pods with mallet or press with flat side of wide knife to "bruise," or crack them open slightly.

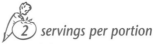

Veggie Lamb Grill

Wonderfully seasoned lamb chops paired with smoky grilled vegetables.
Complementary flavours with a lovely presentation—this recipe is perfect for
a summer barbecue.

Olive (or cooking) oil	3 tbsp.	45 mL
Orange juice	3 tbsp.	45 mL
Dijon mustard	1 tsp.	5 mL
Dried oregano	1/4 tsp.	1 mL
Dried rosemary, crushed	1/4 tsp.	1 mL
Garlic clove, halved	1	1
(or 1/4 tsp., 1 mL, powder)		
Salt	1/4 tsp.	1 mL
Pepper	1/4 tsp.	1 mL
Asian eggplant slices (with peel), cut	12	12
diagonally (about 1/2 inch, 12 mm, slices)		
Zucchini slices (with peel), cut diagonally	12	12
(about 1/2 inch, 12 mm, slices)		
Large red pepper, quartered	1	1
Lamb loin chops (about 3/4 inch,	8	8
2 cm, thick)		
Salt	1/8 tsp.	0.5 mL
Pepper	1/8 tsp.	0.5 mL

Process first 8 ingredients in blender until smooth. Reserve 2 tbsp. (30 mL) in small cup. Transfer remaining orange juice mixture to medium bowl.

Add next 3 ingredients. Toss until coated.

Preheat gas barbecue to medium-high. Sprinkle both sides of chops with salt and pepper. Brush with half of reserved orange juice mixture. Arrange chops and vegetables on greased grill. Close lid. Cook lamb for about 3 minutes per side, brushing occasionally with remaining orange juice mixture, until internal temperature reaches 145°F (63°C) for medium-rare or until desired doneness. Cook vegetables for about 3 minutes per side until tender-crisp. Transfer lamb and vegetables to serving platter. Cover with foil. Let stand for 5 minutes. Serves 4.

1 serving: 330 Calories; 18 g Total Fat (11 g Mono, 1.5 g Poly, 4.5 g Sat); 100 mg Cholesterol;
8 g Carbohydrate; 3 g Fibre; 33 g Protein; 300 mg Sodium

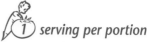
Rhubarb-stuffed Pork

Tart rhubarb, peppery parsnip and spicy ginger add loads of character to tender pork roast. Definitely a company-worthy dish.

Apricot jam	1/4 cup	60 mL
Ground ginger	1/2 tsp.	2 mL
Dried crushed chilies	1/4 tsp.	1 mL
Cooking oil	2 tsp.	10 mL
Chopped onion	3/4 cup	175 mL
Diced parsnip	3/4 cup	175 mL
Finely chopped fresh (or frozen, thawed) rhubarb	2 cups	500 mL
Chopped raisins	1/2 cup	125 mL
Salt	1/4 tsp.	1 mL
Ground cloves, sprinkle		
Unseasoned croutons	1 cup	250 mL
Boneless pork loin roast	3 lbs.	1.4 kg
Salt, sprinkle		
Pepper, sprinkle		

Combine first 3 ingredients in small bowl. Set aside.

Heat cooking oil in large frying pan on medium. Add onion and parsnip. Cook for about 8 minutes, stirring often, until onion is softened.

Add next 4 ingredients. Cook for 5 minutes, stirring occasionally. Transfer to large bowl.

Add croutons. Stir until moistened. Let stand for 10 minutes.

To butterfly roast, cut horizontally lengthwise almost, but not quite through, to other side. Open flat. Place between 2 sheets of plastic wrap. Pound with mallet or rolling pin to 1 inch (2.5 cm) thickness. Spoon rhubarb mixture evenly over cut-side of pork, leaving 1/2 inch (12 mm) edge. Roll up from 1 short edge to enclose filling. Tie with butcher's string.

(continued on next page)

Sprinkle with salt and pepper. Place, seam-side down, on greased wire rack set in medium roasting pan.

Cook, uncovered, in 400°F (200°C) oven for about 30 minutes until starting to brown. Reduce heat to 325°F (160°C). Brush roast with jam mixture. Cook, uncovered, for about 1 hour until internal temperature of pork (not stuffing) reaches 155°F (68°C). Transfer to cutting board. Cover with foil. Let stand for 10 minutes. Internal temperature should rise to at least 160°F (71°C). Remove and discard string. Cut roast into 1/2 inch (12 mm) slices. Serves 8.

1 serving: 590 Calories; 43 g Total Fat (19 g Mono, 4.5 g Poly, 14 g Sat); 120 mg Cholesterol; 23 g Carbohydrate; 2 g Fibre; 28 g Protein; 190 mg Sodium

Pictured on page 53.

 Don't have any leftover chicken or turkey? Start with two boneless, skinless chicken or turkey breast halves (4 – 6 oz., 113 – 117 g, each). Place in large frying pan with 1 cup (250 mL) water or chicken broth. Simmer, covered, for 12 to 14 minuts until no longer pink inside. Drain. Chop. Makes about 2 cups (500 mL) of cooked chicken or turkey.

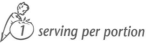

Mac 'n' Cheese Masquerade

*It's a cinch to hide a healthy dose of vegetables in this kid-friendly recipe.
This is one cheesy casserole that's sure to please everyone!*

Water	12 cups	3 L
Salt	1 1/2 tsp.	7 mL
Elbow macaroni	2 cups	500 mL
Sliced carrot	1 cup	250 mL
Broccoli florets	2 cups	500 mL
Frozen peas, thawed	1 cup	250 mL
Lean ground pork	1 lb.	454 g
Chopped onion	1/4 cup	60 mL
Salt	1/4 tsp.	1 mL
2% cottage cheese	1 1/2 cups	375 mL
Herb and garlic cream cheese	1/2 cup	125 mL
Grated Italian cheese blend	1 1/2 cups	375 mL

Combine water and salt in Dutch oven. Bring to a boil. Add pasta. Boil, uncovered, for 4 minutes, stirring occasionally.

Add carrot. Boil for 2 minutes, stirring occasionally. Add broccoli. Boil for 2 minutes, stirring occasionally. Drain, reserving 3/4 cup (175 mL) cooking water. Return pasta and vegetables to same pot.

Add peas. Stir. Cover to keep warm.

Scramble-fry next 3 ingredients in large frying pan on medium-high for about 8 minutes until pork starts to brown. Add to pasta mixture.

Carefully process cottage cheese, cream cheese and reserved cooking water in blender or food processor until smooth (see Safety Tip). Add to pasta mixture. Stir. Transfer to greased 9 x 13 inch (23 x 33 cm) baking dish.

Sprinkle with Italian cheese blend. Bake in 400°F (200°C) oven for about 25 minutes until heated through and golden on top. Serves 8.

1 serving: 310 Calories; 11 g Total Fat (0 g Mono, 0 g Poly, 6 g Sat); 40 mg Cholesterol; 32 g Carbohydrate; 2 g Fibre; 20 g Protein; 510 mg Sodium

Safety Tip: Follow manufacturer's instructions for processing hot liquids.

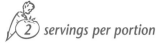 *servings per portion*

Hearty Pork Stew

A colourful stew of nutritious veggies with tender pork and a touch of mustard to round out the flavours. This filling stew is really something special.

All-purpose flour	1/4 cup	60 mL
Dry mustard	2 tsp.	10 mL
Pepper	1/4 tsp.	1 mL
Boneless pork shoulder blade steaks, trimmed of fat, cut into 1 inch (2.5 cm) cubes	1 1/2 lbs.	680 g
Cooking oil	1 tbsp.	15 mL
Prepared chicken broth	3 cups	750 mL
Can of white kidney beans, rinsed and drained	19 oz.	540 mL
Chopped fresh (or frozen) green beans (1 inch, 2.5 cm, pieces)	2 cups	500 mL
Chopped carrot	1 1/2 cups	375 mL
Chopped onion	1 1/2 cups	375 mL
Chopped kale leaves, lightly packed (see Tip, page 131)	3 cups	750 mL
Chopped red pepper	1 1/2 cups	375 mL
Dijon mustard	2 tbsp.	30 mL
White vinegar	1 tbsp.	15 mL
Liquid honey	2 tsp.	10 mL
Salt	1/2 tsp.	2 mL

Combine first 3 ingredients in large resealable freezer bag. Add pork. Seal bag. Toss until coated. Remove pork. Reserve any remaining flour mixture.

Heat cooking oil in Dutch oven on medium-high. Add pork. Cook for about 5 minutes, stirring occasionally, until browned.

Add next 5 ingredients and reserved flour mixture. Stir. Bring to a boil. Reduce heat to medium-low. Simmer, covered, for about 1 hour, stirring occasionally, until pork is tender.

Add remaining 6 ingredients. Stir. Simmer, covered, for about 15 minutes until kale is tender. Makes about 10 cups (2.5 L). Serves 6.

1 serving: 460 Calories; 25 g Total Fat (11 g Mono, 3.5 g Poly, 8 g Sat); 65 mg Cholesterol; 32 g Carbohydrate; 7 g Fibre; 29 g Protein; 1330 mg Sodium

Pictured on page 107.

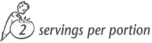

Pork and Sprout Hash

*You'll find tasty Asian flavours with a touch of heat in this interesting mix
containing seasoned pork, sliced Brussels sprouts, potatoes and bean sprouts.*

Rice vinegar	2 tbsp.	30 mL
Soy sauce	2 tbsp.	30 mL
Granulated sugar	4 tsp.	20 mL
Sesame oil (for flavour)	4 tsp.	20 mL
Dried crushed chilies	1/2 tsp.	2 mL
Garlic clove, minced	1	1
(or 1/4 tsp., 1 mL, powder)		
Pork tenderloin, trimmed of fat, halved lengthwise and cut into 1/4 inch (6 mm) slices	1 lb.	454 g
Cooking oil	2 tsp.	10 mL
Cooking oil	2 tsp.	10 mL
Diced peeled potato	2 cups	500 mL
Brussels sprouts (about 6 oz., 170 g), trimmed and halved lengthwise (see Tip, page 105)	1 1/2 cups	375 mL
Fresh bean sprouts	1 cup	250 mL
Roasted sesame seeds	1 tsp.	5 mL

Combine first 6 ingredients in small bowl. Transfer 1 tbsp. (15 mL) to
medium bowl. Add pork. Toss.

Heat first amount of cooking oil in large frying pan on medium-high. Cook
pork, in 2 batches, for about 3 minutes per batch, turning occasionally,
until browned and no longer pink inside. Transfer to plate. Cover to keep
warm. Reduce heat to medium.

Heat second amount of cooking oil in same frying pan. Add potato. Cook,
covered, for about 12 minutes, stirring occasionally, until golden and
tender.

Add Brussels sprouts and remaining rice vinegar mixture. Stir. Cook,
covered, for about 3 minutes, stirring occasionally, until Brussels sprouts
start to soften.

(continued on next page)

Add bean sprouts, sesame seeds and pork. Cook, uncovered, for about 2 minutes, stirring often, until heated through. Makes about 5 cups (1.25 L). Serves 4.

1 serving: 330 Calories; 16 g Total Fat (7 g Mono, 4 g Poly, 3.5 g Sat); 75 mg Cholesterol; 19 g Carbohydrate; 3 g Fibre; 28 g Protein; 530 mg Sodium

Pictured on page 107.

 Select Brussels sprouts that are heavy for their size and bright green with tight leaves. Small heads, about 1 inch (2.5 cm) in diameter, are best. Before cooking, remove any brown leaves and trim the stem ends.

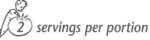

Stuffed Zucchini Boats

A fun presentation. Tender zucchini are stuffed with a tasty mixture of spicy sausage, Asiago and garlic.

Small zucchini, halved lengthwise	4	4
Large egg, fork-beaten	1	1
Fresh bread crumbs (about 2 slices)	1 cup	250 mL
Grated Asiago cheese	1/2 cup	125 mL
Chopped fresh parsley	1 tbsp.	15 mL
(or 3/4 tsp., 4 mL, flakes)		
Garlic clove, minced	1	1
(or 1/4 tsp., 1 mL, powder)		
Hot Italian sausage, casing removed	1/2 lb.	225 g
Olive (or cooking) oil	2 tsp.	10 mL

Scoop out pulp from zucchini halves, leaving 1/4 inch (6 mm) shell (see Note). Arrange shells on greased baking sheet with sides. Chop pulp. Transfer to large bowl.

Add next 5 ingredients. Stir.

Add sausage. Mix well. Spoon into zucchini shells.

Drizzle with olive oil. Cook in 375°F (190°C) oven for about 35 minutes until zucchini is tender and internal temperature reaches 160°F (71°C). Makes 8 stuffed zucchini. Serves 4.

1 serving: 400 Calories; 24 g Total Fat (2.5 g Mono, 1 g Poly, 8 g Sat); 85 mg Cholesterol; 27 g Carbohydrate; 3 g Fibre; 18 g Protein; 840 mg Sodium

Pictured at right.

Note: A melon baller or a round 1/2 tsp. (2 mL) measuring spoon works well for scooping out zucchini pulp.

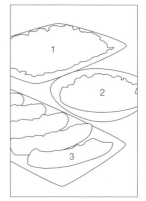

1. Pork and Sprout Hash, page 104
2. Hearty Pork Stew, page 103
3. Stuffed Zucchini Boats, above

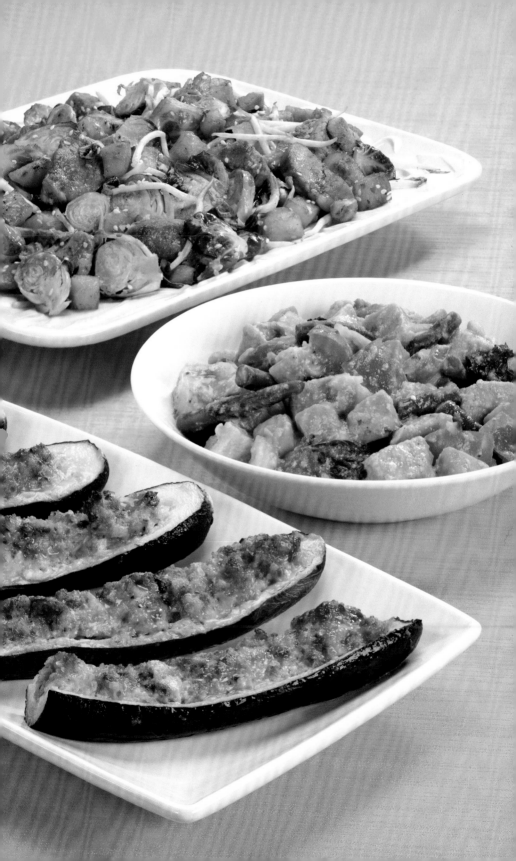

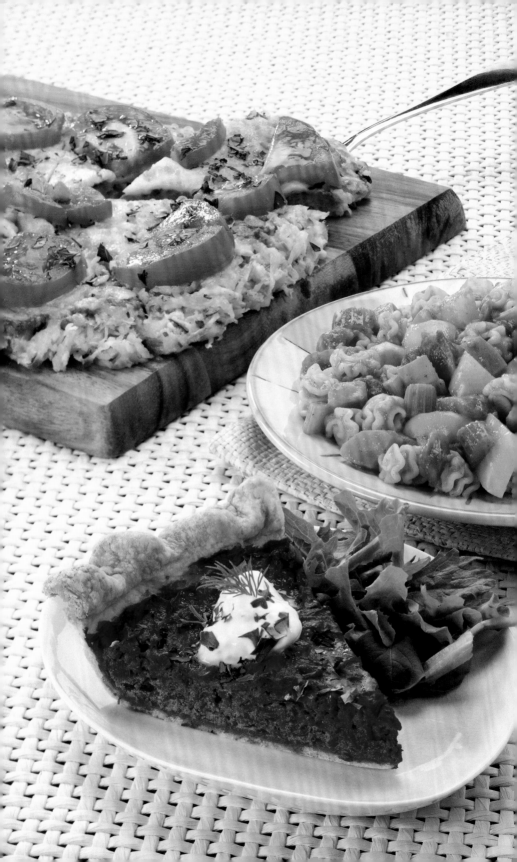

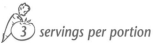

Tenderloin Potato Bake

Yummy tenderloin with a sweet mango glaze, surrounded by potatoes and mushrooms. This mildly seasoned mix is both hearty and satisfying.

Pork tenderloin, trimmed of fat	1 lb.	454 g
Seasoned salt	1/4 tsp.	1 mL
Pepper, sprinkle		
Cooking oil	1 tbsp.	15 mL
Halved fresh white mushrooms	3 cups	750 mL
Chopped peeled potato	2 cups	500 mL
Chopped onion	1 cup	250 mL
Seasoned salt	1/4 tsp.	1 mL
Pepper	1/8 tsp.	0.5 mL
Mango chutney, larger pieces chopped, warmed	2 tbsp.	30 mL

Sprinkle pork with first amounts of seasoned salt and pepper. Heat cooking oil in large frying pan on medium-high. Add pork. Cook for about 5 minutes, turning occasionally, until pork starts to brown. Transfer to greased 9 x 13 inch (23 x 33 cm) baking dish. Reduce heat to medium.

Add next 5 ingredients to same frying pan. Cook for about 8 minutes, stirring often, until onion is softened and liquid is evaporated. Spoon around pork.

Spread chutney over pork. Cook in 350°F (175°C) oven for about 40 minutes until internal temperature of pork reaches 160°F (71°C). Cover with foil. Let stand for 5 minutes. Cut into thin slices. Serve with vegetables. Makes about 2 3/4 cups (675 mL) vegetables. Serves 4.

1 serving: 280 Calories; 10 g Total Fat (4.5 g Mono, 1.5 g Poly, 2.5 g Sat); 75 mg Cholesterol; 21 g Carbohydrate; 2 g Fibre; 27 g Protein; 380 mg Sodium

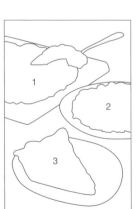

1. Rosti Pizza, page 112
2. Vegetable Radiatore Stew, page 115
3. Borscht Tart, page 111

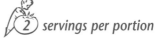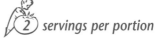 *servings per portion*

Moussaka

This traditional Greek dish makes good use of eggplant. Combined with tender lamb and plenty of cheese, what's not to love? Serve with a Greek salad to continue the dinner theme.

Medium eggplants	2	2
(about 1 1/4 lbs., 560 g, each)		
Cooking oil	2 tbsp.	30 mL
Lean ground lamb	1 lb.	454 g
Chopped onion	1 cup	250 mL
Garlic cloves, minced	2	2
(or 1/2 tsp., 2 mL, powder)		
Can of diced tomatoes, drained	14 oz.	398 mL
Alfredo pasta sauce	1/2 cup	125 mL
Granulated sugar	1/2 tsp.	2 mL
Ground cinnamon	1/4 tsp.	1 mL
Salt	1/4 tsp.	1 mL
Pepper	1/4 tsp.	1 mL
Ground allspice	1/8 tsp.	0.5 mL
Grated mozzarella cheese	1 1/2 cups	375 mL

Cut each eggplant lengthwise into 10 slices, about 1/4 inch (6 mm) each. Discard outside slices. Brush both sides of eggplant slices with cooking oil. Arrange in single layer on greased baking sheets with sides. Broil on top rack in oven for about 6 minutes per side until softened and browned.

Scramble-fry next 3 ingredients in large frying pan on medium-high for about 10 minutes until lamb starts to brown.

Add next 7 ingredients. Heat and stir until boiling. Arrange half of eggplant slices in greased 9 x 13 inch (23 x 33 cm) baking dish. Spread half of lamb mixture evenly over top. Repeat with remaining eggplant slices and lamb mixture.

Sprinkle with cheese. Cover with greased foil. Cook in 350°F (175°C) oven for 45 minutes. Remove and discard foil. Cook for about 15 minutes until golden. Let stand for 10 minutes. Cuts into 8 pieces. Serves 8.

1 serving: 270 Calories; 18 g Total Fat (3 g Mono, 1 g Poly, 9 g Sat); 60 mg Cholesterol; 13 g Carbohydrate; 4 g Fibre; 16 g Protein; 420 mg Sodium

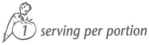
Borscht Tart

Classic borscht flavours served in an unexpected way—this modern take on a traditional favourite packs vegetables into a tart! Surprisingly sweet with nice cayenne pepper heat.

Pastry for 9 inch (23 cm) deep dish pie shell

Cooking oil	1 tsp.	5 mL
Grated peeled beets (see Tip, page 61)	2 cups	500 mL
Chopped onion	1 cup	250 mL
Lemon juice	1 tbsp.	15 mL
Garlic cloves, minced	2	2
(or 1/2 tsp., 2 mL, powder)		
Cayenne pepper	1/4 tsp.	1 mL
Salt	1/4 tsp.	1 mL
Pepper	1/4 tsp.	1 mL
Large eggs, fork-beaten	2	2
Sour cream	1 cup	250 mL
Chopped walnuts, toasted (see Tip, page 38)	1/4 cup	60 mL
Chopped fresh parsley	2 tbsp.	30 mL

Sour cream, for garnish

Roll out pastry on lightly floured surface to 1/8 inch (3 mm) thickness. Line 9 inch (23 cm) deep dish pie plate. Trim, leaving 1/2 inch (12 mm) overhang. Roll under and crimp decorative edge.

Heat cooking oil in large frying pan on medium. Add next 7 ingredients. Cook for about 10 minutes, stirring often, until onion and beets are softened. Let stand for 5 minutes to cool slightly.

Combine next 3 ingredients in medium bowl. Add beet mixture. Stir. Spoon into pie shell. Bake on bottom rack in 375°F (190°C) oven for about 1 hour until knife inserted in centre comes out clean. Let stand for 5 minutes.

Sprinkle with parsley.

Garnish individual servings with sour cream. Cuts into 6 wedges. Serves 6.

1 serving: 320 Calories; 23 g Total Fat (8 g Mono, 6 g Poly, 8 g Sat); 65 mg Cholesterol; 23 g Carbohydrate; 3 g Fibre; 6 g Protein; 310 mg Sodium

Pictured on page 108.

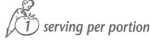

Rosti Pizza

This recipe makes use of some unlikely pizza ingredients. Potato and celery root form the crust of this tasty pizza that's topped with lots of herb flavour and a mild chili heat.

Grated celery root	1 3/4 cups	425 mL
Grated peeled potato	1 3/4 cups	425 mL
Finely chopped onion	1/2 cup	125 mL
Large egg, fork-beaten	1	1
All-purpose flour	1/4 cup	60 mL
Cooking oil	1 tbsp.	15 mL
Dried rosemary, crushed	1/2 tsp.	2 mL
Salt	1/2 tsp.	2 mL
Pepper	1/4 tsp.	1 mL
Cooking oil	2 tbsp.	30 mL
Tomato sauce	1/4 cup	60 mL
Sun-dried tomato pesto	2 tbsp.	30 mL
Dried crushed chilies	1/4 tsp.	1 mL
Grated Italian cheese blend	1 cup	250 mL
Large tomato slices, halved	4	4
Chopped fresh basil	2 tsp.	10 mL

Place first 3 ingredients in fine sieve. Let stand over medium bowl for 15 minutes. Squeeze celery root mixture to remove excess moisture. Transfer to large bowl.

Add next 6 ingredients. Mix well.

Heat 1 tbsp. (15 mL) cooking oil in large non-stick frying pan on medium. Spoon celery root mixture into pan. Press down lightly to cover bottom of pan. Cook for about 10 minutes until bottom is crisp and golden. Slide onto plate. Heat remaining cooking oil in same frying pan. Invert celery root mixture onto another plate. Slide into pan, golden side-up. Cook for about 5 minutes until bottom is crisp and golden.

Combine next 3 ingredients in small bowl. Spread over celery root mixture, almost to edge. Sprinkle with cheese. Broil on centre rack in oven for about 2 minutes until cheese is melted (see Note). Transfer to cutting board.

(continued on next page)

Arrange tomato slices over top. Sprinkle with basil. Cuts into 8 wedges. Serve immediately. Serves 4.

1 serving: 330 Calories; 19 g Total Fat (7 g Mono, 3 g Poly, 4.5 g Sat); 55 mg Cholesterol; 28 g Carbohydrate; 3 g Fibre; 11 g Protein; 660 mg Sodium

Pictured on page 108.

Note: When baking or broiling food in a frying pan with a handle that isn't ovenproof, wrap the handle in foil and keep it to the front of the oven, away from the element.

2 servings per portion

Barley-stuffed Peppers

Stuffed peppers always make a bold statement. Tomatoey barley and veggies are conveniently packed into fresh bell peppers.

Cooking oil	1 tbsp.	15 mL
Sliced celery	1 1/2 cups	375 mL
Chopped onion	1 cup	250 mL
Pearl barley	1/2 cup	125 mL
Can of diced tomatoes (with juice)	14 oz.	398 mL
Vegetable cocktail juice	1 1/2 cups	375 mL
Dried basil	1/2 tsp.	2 mL
Dried oregano	1/2 tsp.	2 mL
Granulated sugar	1/2 tsp.	2 mL
Dried thyme	1/4 tsp.	1 mL
Salt	1/4 tsp.	1 mL
Pepper	1/4 tsp.	1 mL
Cayenne pepper, sprinkle (optional)		
Large green peppers, halved lengthwise	3	3

Heat cooking oil in large saucepan on medium. Add celery and onion. Cook for about 8 minutes, stirring often, until onion is softened.

Add barley. Stir. Add next 9 ingredients. Stir. Bring to a boil. Reduce heat to medium-low. Simmer, covered, for about 40 minutes, stirring occasionally, until barley is tender.

Place pepper halves, cut-side up, in greased 9 x 13 inch (23 x 33 cm) baking dish. Fill with barley mixture. Cook, covered, in 400°F (200°C) oven for 25 to 30 minutes until green peppers are tender-crisp. Serves 6.

1 serving: 120 Calories; 3 g Total Fat (1.5 g Mono, 0.5 g Poly, 0 g Sat); 0 mg Cholesterol; 21 g Carbohydrate; 5 g Fibre; 4 g Protein; 460 mg Sodium

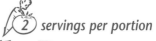

Vietnamese Portobello Burgers

A unique vegetarian main course with a Vietnamese-inspired topping and a portobello mushroom in place of a bun.

Granulated sugar	3 tbsp.	45 mL
Rice vinegar	1/3 cup	75 mL
Coleslaw mix	1 cup	250 mL
Thinly sliced onion	1/4 cup	60 mL
Chopped pickled pepper rings	3 tbsp.	45 mL
Can of lentils, rinsed and drained	19 oz.	540 mL
Chopped carrot	1/4 cup	60 mL
Garlic clove, minced	1	1
(or 1/4 tsp., 1 mL, powder)		
Salt	1/4 tsp.	1 mL
Pepper	1/4 tsp.	1 mL
Large egg, fork-beaten	1	1
Quick-cooking rolled oats	1/2 cup	125 mL
Portobello mushrooms (about 4 inch, 10 cm, diameter), stems and gills removed (see Tip, page 136)	4	4
Sesame oil (for flavour)	1 tbsp.	15 mL
Chopped fresh cilantro (or parsley)	1 tbsp.	15 mL

Stir sugar into rice vinegar in small bowl until dissolved.

Add next 3 ingredients. Stir. Marinate, covered, in refrigerator for 1 hour. Drain. Squeeze to remove excess moisture. Return to same small bowl.

Put next 5 ingredients into food processor. Pulse with on/off motion until lentils are mashed but not puréed. Transfer to medium bowl.

Add egg and oats. Mix well. Divide into 4 equal portions. Shape into 4 inch (10 cm) patties.

Press patties firmly into mushrooms. Brush both sides with sesame oil. Preheat gas barbecue to medium. Place mushrooms, patty-side down, on well-greased grill. Close lid. Cook for about 8 minutes until internal temperature of patty reaches 165°F (74°C). Turn. Close lid. Cook for about 4 minutes until mushroom is tender and browned.

(continued on next page)

Top with coleslaw mixture. Sprinkle with cilantro. Makes 4 burgers. Serves 4.

1 serving: 290 Calories; 6 g Total Fat (2 g Mono, 2 g Poly, 1 g Sat); 35 mg Cholesterol;
47 g Carbohydrate; 8 g Fibre; 13 g Protein; 480 mg Sodium

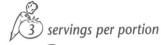 *servings per portion*

Vegetable Radiatore Stew

North African spices accent deliciously healthy veggies in this hearty pasta
stew. Serve with a loaf of multigrain bread to soak up the sauce.

Cooking oil	2 tsp.	10 mL
Chopped purple-topped turnip	2 cups	500 mL
Chopped carrot	1 1/2 cups	375 mL
Chopped celery	1 cup	250 mL
Chopped onion	1 cup	250 mL
Ground cumin	1 tsp.	5 mL
Ground ginger	1 tsp.	5 mL
Garlic cloves, minced	2	2
(or 1/2 tsp., 2 mL, powder)		
Ground cinnamon	1/4 tsp.	1 mL
Salt	1/2 tsp.	2 mL
Pepper	1/4 tsp.	1 mL
Can of diced tomatoes (with juice)	28 oz.	796 mL
Prepared vegetable broth	2 cups	500 mL
Granulated sugar	1/2 tsp.	2 mL
Radiatore pasta	2 cups	500 mL
Chopped yellow pepper	1 cup	250 mL

Heat cooking oil in Dutch oven on medium. Add next 10 ingredients. Cook for about 10 minutes, stirring often, until onion is softened.

Add next 3 ingredients. Stir. Bring to a boil.

Add pasta. Stir. Reduce heat to medium-low. Cook, covered, for 5 minutes, stirring occasionally.

Add yellow pepper. Stir. Cook, uncovered, for about 5 minutes, stirring occasionally, until pasta is tender but firm. Makes about 8 1/2 cups (2.1 L). Serves 4.

1 serving: 250 Calories; 3.5 g Total Fat (1.5 g Mono, 0.5 g Poly, 0 g Sat); 0 mg Cholesterol;
50 g Carbohydrate; 5 g Fibre; 8 g Protein; 1220 mg Sodium

Pictured on page 108.

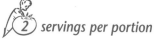
Spinach Pesto Primavera

You'll want to use the freshest seasonal vegetables for this dish. The leftover pesto can be stored in the refrigerator for up to 3 days.

SPINACH PESTO

Fresh basil leaves, lightly packed	1 cup	250 mL
Fresh spinach leaves, lightly packed	1 cup	250 mL
Olive oil	1/4 cup	60 mL
Pine nuts, toasted (see Tip, page 38)	1/4 cup	60 mL
Garlic cloves	3	3
Salt	1/4 tsp.	1 mL
Grated Parmesan cheese	1/2 cup	125 mL

PASTA PRIMAVERA

Linguine	12 oz.	340 g
Butter	1/4 cup	60 mL
Chopped green pepper	1/2 cup	125 mL
Chopped red pepper	1/2 cup	125 mL
Chopped orange pepper	1/2 cup	125 mL
Chopped yellow pepper	1/2 cup	125 mL
Sliced fresh white mushrooms	1/2 cup	125 mL
Grape tomatoes	1 cup	250 mL
Pitted kalamata olives	1/2 cup	125 mL
Grated Parmesan cheese	1/4 cup	60 mL
Pine nuts	1/4 cup	60 mL
Chopped fresh basil, for garnish (optional)		

Spinach Pesto: Process first 6 ingredients in blender until smooth. Transfer to small bowl. Add cheese. Stir well. Makes about 1 cup (250 mL) pesto.

Pasta Primavera: Cook pasta according to package directions. Drain.

Melt butter in large saucepan on medium. Add next 5 ingredients. Cook for 3 to 4 minutes until tender.

Add 1/2 cup (125 mL) Spinach Pesto. Cook for 3 minutes. Add next 3 ingredients. Cook for 5 minutes. Add linguine and toss until coated. Remove from heat.

(continued on next page)

Sprinkle with pine nuts and basil. Serves 4.

1 serving: 410 Calories; 38 g Total Fat (16 g Mono, 6 g Poly, 11 g Sat); 40 mg Cholesterol; 42 g Carbohydrate; 6 g Fibre; 19 g Protein; 860 mg Sodium

Pictured on front cover.

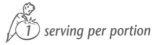 *serving per portion*

Spicy Beans and Rice

This inviting blend of brown rice, black beans and red peppers has great texture and just the right amount of chili spice.

Can of black beans, rinsed and drained	19 oz.	540 mL
Diced red pepper	2 cups	500 mL
Long-grain brown rice	1 1/2 cups	375 mL
Finely chopped celery	1 cup	250 mL
Finely chopped onion	1 cup	250 mL
Dried crushed chilies	1/2 tsp.	2 mL
Dried thyme	1/2 tsp.	2 mL
Salt	1/2 tsp.	2 mL
Pepper	1/4 tsp.	1 mL
Ground allspice	1/8 tsp.	0.5 mL
Prepared vegetable broth	3 1/2 cups	875 mL
Chopped fresh cilantro (or parsley)	1 tbsp.	15 mL

Combine first 10 ingredients in large bowl. Spread evenly in greased 9 x 13 inch (23 x 33 cm) baking dish.

Add broth. Stir. Cook, covered, in 400°F (200°C) oven for about 1 hour, stirring at halftime, until rice is tender. Let stand, covered, for about 10 minutes until liquid is absorbed.

Sprinkle with cilantro. Stir. Makes about 10 cups (2.5 L). Serves 6.

1 serving: 290 Calories; 2.5 g Total Fat (0 g Mono, 0 g Poly, 0 g Sat); 0 mg Cholesterol; 62 g Carbohydrate; 9 g Fibre; 10 g Protein; 680 mg Sodium

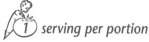

Spaghetti Lasagna

The "spaghetti" in this lasagna is spaghetti squash. Cheese, alfredo sauce and creamy mushrooms make this lasagna delicious and broadly appealing.

Cooking oil	1 tsp.	5 mL
Sliced fresh brown (or white) mushrooms	2 cups	500 mL
Chopped onion	1 cup	250 mL
Alfredo pasta sauce	2 cups	500 mL
Water	1/2 cup	125 mL
Pepper	1/2 tsp.	2 mL
Spaghetti squash	2 1/2 lbs.	1.1 kg
Water	2 tbsp.	30 mL
Basil pesto	1 tbsp.	15 mL
Oven-ready lasagna noodles	8	8
Grated mozzarella cheese	1 cup	250 mL

Heat cooking oil in medium saucepan on medium. Add mushrooms and onion. Cook for about 10 minutes, stirring often, until onion is softened.

Add next 3 ingredients. Stir.

Cut squash in half lengthwise. Remove seeds. Place, cut-side down, in large ungreased microwave-safe 3 quart (3 L) casserole. Add water. Microwave, covered, on high for about 15 minutes until tender (see Tip, page 119). Drain. Let stand until cool enough to handle. Shred squash pulp with fork. Separate into strands. Transfer to medium bowl. Add pesto. Stir. Discard shells.

To assemble, layer ingredients in greased 9 x 13 inch (23 x 33 cm) baking dish as follows:

1. 1 cup (250 mL) mushroom mixture
2. 4 lasagna noodles
3. Half of squash mixture
4. 1 cup (250 mL) mushroom mixture
5. 4 lasagna noodles
6. Remaining squash mixture
7. Remaining mushroom mixture

(continued on next page)

Sprinkle with cheese. Cover with greased foil. Bake in 350°F (175°C) oven for about 50 minutes until noodles are tender. Carefully remove foil. Bake for about 15 minutes until cheese is golden. Let stand for 10 minutes. Cuts into 8 pieces. Serves 8.

1 serving: 260 Calories; 13 g Total Fat (1.5 g Mono, 0.5 g Poly, 7 g Sat); 40 mg Cholesterol; 29 g Carbohydrate; 2 g Fibre; 11 g Protein; 380 mg Sodium

 tip The microwaves used in our test kitchen are 900 watts—but microwaves are sold in many different powers. You should be able to find the wattage of yours by opening the door and looking for the mandatory label. If your microwave is more than 900 watts, you may need to reduce the cooking time. If it's less than 900 watts, you'll probably need to increase the cooking time.

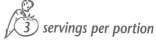

Caramelized Fennel Fusilli

A simple pasta dish with lovely herbs, sweet fennel and bright bites of tomato.
Serve with a sprinkle of Parmesan cheese.

Butter (or hard margarine)	2 tbsp.	30 mL
Thinly sliced fennel bulb (white part only)	4 cups	1 L
Sliced onion	2 cups	500 mL
Fennel seed	1/2 tsp.	2 mL
Salt	1/4 tsp.	1 mL
Prepared vegetable broth	1/3 cup	75 mL
White wine vinegar	1 tbsp.	15 mL
Water	12 cups	3 L
Salt	1 1/2 tsp.	7 mL
Fusilli pasta	4 cups	1 L
Diced tomato	1/2 cup	125 mL
Slivered almonds, toasted (see Tip, page 38)	1/4 cup	60 mL
Chopped fresh basil	1 tbsp.	15 mL
Chopped fresh thyme	1 tsp.	5 mL
Pepper	1/8 tsp.	0.5 mL

Melt butter in large frying pan on medium. Add next 4 ingredients. Stir. Cook, covered, for about 10 minutes until fennel bulb is softened. Stir. Cook, uncovered, for 15 to 20 minutes, stirring occasionally, until onion and fennel bulb are caramelized.

Add broth and vinegar. Cook for about 3 minutes, stirring occasionally, until liquid is evaporated.

Combine water and salt in Dutch oven. Bring to a boil. Add pasta. Boil, uncovered, for 7 to 9 minutes, stirring occasionally, until tender but firm. Drain, reserving 1/2 cup (125 mL) cooking water. Return pasta to same pot.

Add remaining 5 ingredients, fennel mixture and reserved cooking water. Stir. Makes about 7 1/2 cups (1.9 L). Serves 4.

1 serving: 500 Calories; 12 g Total Fat (4 g Mono, 1.5 g Poly, 4 g Sat); 15 mg Cholesterol; 84 g Carbohydrate; 9 g Fibre; 16 g Protein; 330 mg Sodium

Pictured on page 125.

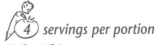

"Okra Dokey" Chili

A chunky vegetable chili, with okra lending a unique look and feel that's reminiscent of gumbo.

Cooking oil	1 tbsp.	15 mL
Chopped onion	1 cup	250 mL
Chopped celery	1/2 cup	125 mL
Cajun seasoning	1 tbsp.	15 mL
Chili powder	1 tbsp.	15 mL
Ground cumin	1 tsp.	5 mL
Garlic clove, minced	1	1
(or 1/4 tsp., 1 mL, powder)		
Sliced fresh (or frozen, thawed) okra	3 cups	750 mL
(about 1/2 inch, 12 mm, slices)		
Can of mixed beans, rinsed and drained	19 oz.	540 mL
Can of diced tomatoes (with juice)	14 oz.	398 mL
Chopped peeled potato	1 1/2 cups	375 mL
Chopped green pepper	1 cup	250 mL
Fresh (or frozen, thawed) kernel corn	1/2 cup	125 mL
Prepared vegetable broth	1/2 cup	125 mL
Can of diced green chilies	4 oz.	113 g
Brown sugar, packed	2 tsp.	10 mL

Heat cooking oil in Dutch oven on medium. Add onion and celery. Cook for about 5 minutes, stirring often, until celery starts to soften.

Add next 4 ingredients. Heat and stir for about 1 minute until garlic is fragrant.

Add remaining 9 ingredients. Stir. Bring to a boil. Reduce heat to medium. Cook, covered, for about 45 minutes, stirring occasionally, until potato is tender. Makes about 7 1/2 cups (1.9 L). Serves 4.

1 serving: 270 Calories; 4 g Total Fat (2 g Mono, 1 g Poly, 0 g Sat); 0 mg Cholesterol; 49 g Carbohydrate; 12 g Fibre; 12 g Protein; 1820 mg Sodium

Pictured on page 125.

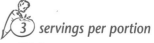

Spinach Cheese Pie

Spanokopita flavours abound in this appetizing pie. Buttery phyllo hides a cheesy spinach filling for a lovely and satisfying combination.

Cooking oil	2 tsp.	10 mL
Chopped onion	1 cup	250 mL
Large eggs, fork-beaten	2	2
Boxes of frozen chopped spinach (10 oz., 300 g, each), thawed and squeezed dry	2	2
Crumbled feta cheese	1 cup	250 mL
Ricotta cheese	3/4 cup	175 mL
Chopped fresh dill (or 2 1/4 tsp., 11 mL, dried)	3 tbsp.	45 mL
Pepper	1/4 tsp.	1 mL
Phyllo pastry sheets, thawed according to package directions	10	10
Cooking spray		
Fine dry bread crumbs	9 tsp.	45 mL

Heat cooking oil in medium frying pan on medium. Add onion. Cook for about 5 minutes, stirring often, until softened. Transfer to large bowl.

Add next 6 ingredients. Stir.

Place 1 pastry sheet on work surface. Cover remaining sheets with damp towel to prevent drying. Spray with cooking spray. Sprinkle with 1 tsp. (5 mL) bread crumbs. Fold into thirds lengthwise to make a 4 inch (10 cm) strip. Repeat with 7 more pastry sheets, cooking spray and bread crumbs. Place 1 pastry strip in greased 9 inch (23 cm) deep dish pie plate, allowing ends of strip to hang over edge. Place second strip over first, at an angle and slightly overlapping. Repeat with remaining pastry strips until entire pie plate is covered (see Diagram 1). Gently press pastry to fit in pie plate, forming crust. Spray with cooking spray. Fill with spinach mixture (see Diagram 2). Spread evenly. Place 1 pastry sheet on work surface. Spray with cooking spray. Sprinkle with 1 tsp. (5 mL) bread crumbs. Cover with remaining pastry sheet. Bunch up loosely. Place over spinach mixture. Bunch overhanging pastry toward centre of pie to cover. Spray with cooking spray. Bake on bottom rack in 350°F (175°C) oven for about 65 minutes until pastry is browned and internal temperature reaches 165°F (74°C). Let stand on wire rack for 10 minutes. Cuts into 6 wedges. Serves 6.

(continued on next page)

1 serving: 340 Calories; 13 g Total Fat (3.5 g Mono, 1 g Poly, 7 g Sat); 80 mg Cholesterol; 37 g Carbohydrate; 6 g Fibre; 19 g Protein; 950 mg Sodium

Pictured on page 125.

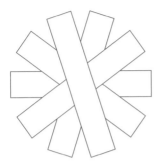

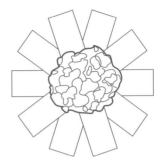

Diagram 1   Diagram 2

HELPFUL HINTS

There are plenty of tricks when it comes to eating vegetables that will save you time and encourage you and your family to eat the recommended daily amount. For example, wash lettuce as soon as you bring it home and wrap it in tea towels—that way it will take no time at all to make a salad come dinnertime. Keep chopped up bell peppers, baby carrots and snap peas in baggies in the fridge—they make a great afternoon or on-the-go snack. Store tomatoes at room temperature for maximum flavour and freshness. Get in the habit of adding vegetables to your everyday staples, whether that's lettuce and cucumber slices on your sandwich or peas in your macaroni casserole.

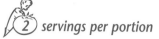

Veggie Tagine

Fruit and vegetable goodness are front and centre in this sweet and tangy tagine. Serve over quinoa or couscous with a dollop of plain yogurt.

Cooking oil	2 tsp.	10 mL
Chopped carrot	1 cup	250 mL
Chopped onion	1 cup	250 mL
Chopped peeled potato	1 cup	250 mL
Cans of chickpeas (garbanzo beans), 19 oz. (540 mL) each, rinsed and drained	2	2
Can of diced tomatoes (with juice)	28 oz.	796 mL
Can of pure pumpkin (no spices)	14 oz.	398 mL
Prepared vegetable broth	1 cup	250 mL
Finely chopped pitted prunes	1/2 cup	125 mL
Finely chopped dried apricot	1/4 cup	60 mL
Ground cumin	1 1/2 tsp.	7 mL
Garlic powder	1/4 tsp.	1 mL
Ground cinnamon	1/4 tsp.	1 mL
Salt	1/4 tsp.	1 mL
Cayenne pepper	1/8 tsp.	0.5 mL

Heat cooking oil in Dutch oven on medium. Add next 3 ingredients. Cook for about 12 minutes, stirring often, until carrot starts to soften.

Add remaining 11 ingredients. Stir. Bring to a boil. Reduce heat to medium-low. Simmer, covered, for about 1 hour until carrot is tender. Makes about 9 1/2 cups (2.4 L). Serves 6.

1 serving: 240 Calories; 3.5 g Total Fat (1 g Mono, 0 g Poly, 0 g Sat); 0 mg Cholesterol; 47 g Carbohydrate; 10 g Fibre; 9 g Protein; 890 mg Sodium

1. Caramelized Fennel Fusilli, page 120
2. "Okra Dokey" Chili, page 121
3. Spinach Cheese Pie, page 122

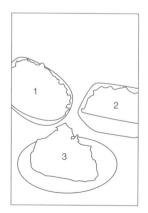

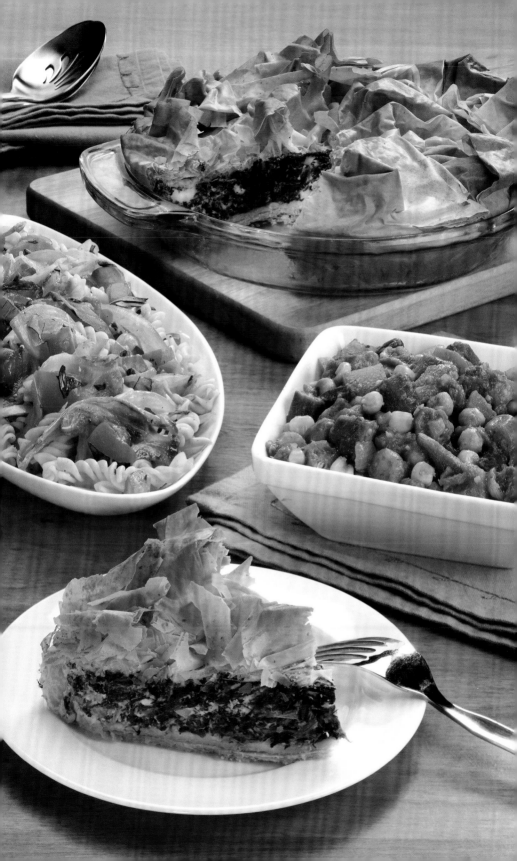

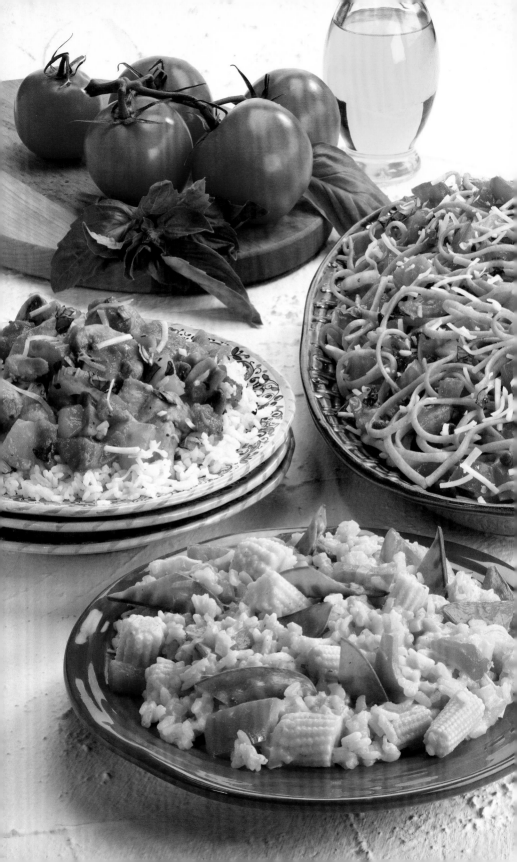

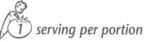

Bruschetta Linguine

Lovely, fresh flavours of tomato, basil and capers pair with whole-wheat pasta. This dish not only tastes good, but is also good for you! Use ripe tomatoes for best results.

Water	12 cups	3 L
Salt	1 1/2 tsp.	7 mL
Whole-wheat linguine	12 oz.	340 g
Diced tomato	4 cups	1 L
Chopped fresh basil	1/2 cup	125 mL
Finely chopped onion	1/2 cup	125 mL
Capers (optional)	1/4 cup	60 mL
Olive oil	2 tbsp.	30 mL
Balsamic vinegar	1 tbsp.	15 mL
Garlic clove, minced,	1	1
(or 1/4 tsp., 1 mL, powder)		
Grated Asiago cheese	1/4 cup	60 mL

Combine water and salt in Dutch oven. Bring to a boil. Add pasta. Boil, uncovered, for 9 to 11 minutes, stirring occasionally, until tender but firm. Drain. Return to same pot.

Add next 7 ingredients. Toss.

Sprinkle with cheese. Makes about 9 1/2 cups (2.4 L). Serves 6.

1 serving: 290 Calories; 10 g Total Fat (3.5 g Mono, 0.5 g Poly, 2 g Sat); trace Cholesterol; 42 g Carbohydrate; 9 g Fibre; 11 g Protein; 60 mg Sodium

Pictured at left.

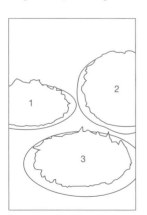

1. Turkey Cacciatore, page 83
2. Bruschetta Linguine, above
3. Curried Coconut Risotto, page 128

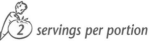
Curried Coconut Risotto

Rich and creamy coconut risotto with yellow curry and satisfying bites tender-crisp vegetables.

Prepared vegetable broth	4 1/2 cups	1.1 L
Can of coconut milk	14 oz.	398 mL
Cooking oil	1 tbsp.	15 mL
Sliced leek (white part only)	1 1/2 cups	375 mL
Curry powder	1 tbsp.	15 mL
Arborio rice	1 1/2 cups	375 mL
Lime juice	2 tbsp.	30 mL
Brown sugar, packed	1 tbsp.	15 mL
Finely grated ginger root	1 tbsp.	15 mL
(or 3/4 tsp., 4 mL, ground ginger)		
Garlic cloves, minced	2	2
(or 1/2 tsp., 2 mL, powder)		
Can of cut baby corn, drained	14 oz.	398 mL
Diagonally sliced trimmed snow peas	1 cup	250 mL
Chopped red pepper	1/2 cup	125 mL

Bring broth and coconut milk to a boil in medium saucepan. Reduce heat to low. Cover to keep hot.

Heat cooking oil in large saucepan on medium. Add leek and curry powder. Cook for about 5 minutes, stirring often, until leek is softened.

Add next 5 ingredients. Heat and stir for about 1 minute until rice is coated and garlic is fragrant. Add 1 cup (250 mL) of hot broth mixture, stirring constantly until broth mixture is absorbed. Repeat with remaining broth mixture, 1 cup (250 mL) at a time, until broth mixture is absorbed and rice is tender and creamy.

Add remaining 3 ingredients. Stir. Let stand, covered, for 5 minutes. Makes about 7 1/4 cups (1.8 L). Serves 4.

1 serving: 580 Calories; 25 g Total Fat (3 g Mono, 1 g Poly, 19 g Sat); 0 mg Cholesterol; 82 g Carbohydrate; 4 g Fibre; 10 g Protein; 900 mg Sodium

Pictured on page 126.

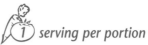

Triple-root Gratin

Find a satisfying array of root vegetables—potato, parsnip and celery—in this rich and cheesy gratin.

Butter (or hard margarine)	2 tbsp.	30 mL
Chopped onion	1/2 cup	125 mL
Garlic clove, minced	1	1
(or 1/4 tsp., 1 mL, powder)		
All-purpose flour	2 tbsp.	30 mL
Salt	1/4 tsp.	1 mL
Pepper	1/4 tsp.	1 mL
Prepared chicken broth	2 cups	500 mL
Grated Gruyère cheese	1 cup	250 mL
Prepared horseradish	1 1/2 tsp.	7 mL
Thinly sliced peeled baking potato (see Note)	2 cups	500 mL
Thinly sliced celery root (see Note)	1 cup	250 mL
Thinly sliced parsnip (see Note)	1 cup	250 mL
Grated Gruyère cheese	1/2 cup	125 mL

Melt butter in medium saucepan on medium. Add onion and garlic. Cook for about 5 minutes, stirring often, until onion is softened.

Add next 3 ingredients. Heat and stir for 1 minute. Slowly add broth, stirring constantly until smooth. Heat and stir until boiling and thickened. Remove from heat.

Add first amount of cheese and horseradish. Stir until cheese is melted.

Combine next 3 ingredients and cheese mixture in large bowl. Spoon into greased shallow 2 quart (2 L) casserole.

Sprinkle second amount of cheese over top. Cook, covered, in 350°F (175°C) oven for about 1 hour until vegetables are tender. Remove cover. Cook for about 5 minutes until golden. Let stand for 5 minutes. Serves 6.

1 serving: 190 Calories; 10 g Total Fat (3 g Mono, 0.5 g Poly, 6 g Sat); 30 mg Cholesterol; 19 g Carbohydrate; 3 g Fibre; 8 g Protein; 390 mg Sodium

Note: Evenly sliced vegetables are one of the secrets to a good gratin. Use a mandoline slicer or food processor to ensure equal slices.

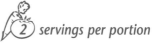

Broccoli Curry

Ease your family into the idea of eating curry with this mild beginner dish.
Heat the sauce while the broccoli is cooking for a quick and convenient
weeknight side.

Broccoli florets	6 cups	1.5 L
Can of condensed cream of celery soup	10 oz.	284 mL
Sour cream	1/4 cup	60 mL
Curry powder	1 tsp.	5 mL
Pepper	1/8 tsp.	0.5 mL

Pour water into large saucepan until about 1 inch (2.5 cm) deep. Add broccoli. Cover. Bring to a boil. Reduce heat to medium. Boil gently for about 4 minutes until bright green and tender-crisp. Drain. Transfer to serving bowl. Cover to keep warm.

Combine remaining 4 ingredients in small saucepan. Heat and stir on medium until hot, but not boiling. Pour over broccoli. Makes about 6 cups (1.5 L). Serves 6.

1 serving: 80 Calories; 4.5 g Total Fat (1 g Mono, 1.5 g Poly, 2 g Sat); 10 mg Cholesterol; 8 g Carbohydrate; 0 g Fibre; 3 g Protein; 420 mg Sodium

 servings per portion

Lemon Dill Potatoes

A simple cooking method brings out the best in baby potatoes. A versatile side
for pairing with grilled or roast meats.

Baby potatoes, larger ones halved	1 1/2 lbs.	680 g
Olive oil	1 tbsp.	15 mL
Chopped fresh dill	2 tsp.	10 mL
(or 1/2 tsp., 2 mL, dried)		
Grated onion	2 tsp.	10 mL
Lemon juice	2 tsp.	10 mL
Dijon mustard	1/2 tsp.	2 mL
Salt	1/2 tsp.	2 mL
Coarsely ground pepper	1/2 tsp.	2 mL

(continued on next page)

Place potatoes in steamer basket set over rapidly boiling water in large saucepan or Dutch oven. Cover. Steam for about 15 minutes, adding more boiling water to pot if necessary, until tender.

Combine remaining 7 ingredients in large bowl. Add potatoes. Toss. Makes about 4 cups (1 L). Serves 4.

1 serving: 170 Calories; 3.5 g Total Fat (2.5 g Mono, 0 g Poly, 0 g Sat); 0 mg Cholesterol; 31 g Carbohydrate; 2 g Fibre; 4 g Protein; 260 mg Sodium

────────────── 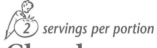 *servings per portion*

Raspberry Ruby Chard

Colourful ruby chard gets a little assistance from tangy raspberry dressing. This lovely dish goes great with roasted meats.

Ruby chard	1 lb.	454 g
Cooking oil	1 tsp.	5 mL
Salt, sprinkle		
Pepper, sprinkle		
Raspberry vinaigrette dressing	4 tsp.	20 mL

Remove chard stems from leaves (see Tip, below). Slice leaves into 2 inch (5 cm) strips. Slice stems into 1 1/2 inch (4 cm) pieces.

Heat cooking oil in Dutch oven on medium. Add stems. Sprinkle with salt and pepper. Cook for about 5 minutes, stirring occasionally, until tender-crisp. Add leaves. Cook, covered, for about 4 minutes, stirring once, until leaves are wilted.

Add dressing. Stir. Makes about 4 cups (1 L). Serves 4.

1 serving: 45 Calories; 2.5 g Total Fat (0.5 g Mono, 0 g Poly, 0 g Sat); 0 mg Cholesterol; 5 g Carbohydrate; 2 g Fibre; 2 g Protein; 270 mg Sodium

Pictured on page 90.

 tip To remove the centre rib from lettuce, kale or Swiss chard, fold the leaf in half along the rib and then cut along the length of the rib.

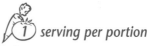

Veggie Fried Rice

Asian veggies make this fried rice both colourful and delicious. The inclusion of edamame beans pumps up the protein and also makes this side a suitable vegetarian main course.

Cooking oil	1 tbsp.	15 mL
Can of cut baby corn, drained	14 oz.	398 mL
Halved trimmed snow peas	1 cup	250 mL
Finely chopped carrot	1/2 cup	125 mL
Frozen shelled edamame (soybeans)	1/2 cup	125 mL
Sliced green onion	1/4 cup	60 mL
Soy sauce	3 tbsp.	45 mL
Ground ginger	1 tsp.	5 mL
Garlic powder	1/2 tsp.	2 mL
Salt	1/8 tsp.	0.5 mL
Cold cooked long-grain white rice (about 1 cup, 250 mL, uncooked)	3 cups	750 mL

Heat large frying pan or wok on medium-high until very hot. Add cooking oil. Add next 4 ingredients. Stir-fry for about 2 minutes until carrot is tender-crisp.

Add next 5 ingredients. Stir-fry for 1 minute.

Add rice. Stir-fry for about 3 minutes until rice is coated and heated through.

Makes about 6 cups (1.5 L). Serves 6.

1 serving: 160 Calories; 3 g Total Fat (1.5 g Mono, 0.5 g Poly, 0 g Sat); 0 mg Cholesterol; 27 g Carbohydrate; 3 g Fibre; 6 g Protein; 670 mg Sodium

Pictured on page 90.

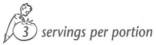

Fragrant Herbed Vegetables

Roasting vegetables brings out their natural sweetness. Butter and herbs round out the flavours for this extraordinarily simple side.

Diagonally sliced carrot (about 1/2 inch, 12 mm, slices)	3 cups	750 mL
Sliced onion (about 1/2 inch, 12 mm, slices)	1 cup	250 mL
Cooking oil	2 tbsp.	30 mL
Salt	1/4 tsp.	1 mL
Coarsely ground pepper	1/2 tsp.	2 mL
Diagonally sliced parsnip (about 1/2 inch, 12 mm, slices)	3 cups	750 mL
Garlic clove, thinly sliced	1	1
Butter (or hard margarine), softened	1 tbsp.	15 mL
Chopped fresh chives (or green onion)	1 tbsp.	15 mL
Chopped fresh rosemary	1/2 tsp.	2 mL
Chopped fresh thyme	1/2 tsp.	2 mL

Toss first 5 ingredients in large bowl until coated. Spread in single layer in greased 9 x 13 inch (23 x 33 cm) baking dish. Cook in 450°F (230°C) oven for 15 minutes.

Add parsnip and garlic. Stir. Cook for about 30 minutes, stirring at halftime, until vegetables are tender and browned. Transfer to serving bowl.

Combine remaining 4 ingredients in small cup. Add to vegetable mixture. Stir. Makes about 4 cups (1 L). Serves 4.

1 serving: 200 Calories; 10 g Total Fat (5 g Mono, 2 g Poly, 2.5 g Sat); 10 mg Cholesterol; 28 g Carbohydrate; 7 g Fibre; 2 g Protein; 190 mg Sodium

Pictured on page 90.

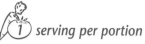 *serving per portion*

Grilled Asparagus

Crispy, buttery asparagus with a delicious smoky flavour from grilling.
A hint of lemon completes the experience.

Butter (or hard margarine), melted	3 tbsp.	45 mL
Grated lemon zest	1/4 tsp.	1 mL
Ground ginger	1/4 tsp.	1 mL
Pepper	1/8 tsp.	0.5 mL
Fresh asparagus, trimmed of tough ends	1 lb.	454 g

Combine first 4 ingredients in small cup.

Brush over asparagus. Preheat gas barbecue to medium. Place asparagus crosswise on greased grill. Close lid. Cook for about 5 minutes, turning at halftime and brushing with any remaining butter mixture, until tender-crisp. Serves 6.

1 serving: 60 Calories; 6 g Total Fat (1.5 g Mono, 0 g Poly, 3.5 g Sat); 15 mg Cholesterol; 2 g Carbohydrate; 1 g Fibre; 1 g Protein; 40 mg Sodium

Pictured on page 53.

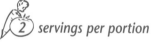 *servings per portion*

Spiced Sweet Potatoes

Glazed sweet potatoes are paired with a nice spice blend for a unique side dish that you won't soon forget.

Cubed peeled orange-fleshed sweet potato (1 inch, 2.5 cm, pieces)	4 cups	1 L
Brown sugar, packed	3 tbsp.	45 mL
Butter (or hard margarine), softened	2 tbsp.	30 mL
Ground cinnamon	1/4 tsp.	1 mL
Salt	1/4 tsp.	1 mL
Cayenne pepper	1/8 tsp.	0.5 mL
Ground nutmeg	1/8 tsp.	0.5 mL

Place sweet potato in greased 2 quart (2 L) casserole. Cook, covered, in 375°F (190°C) oven for about 30 minutes until almost tender.

(continued on next page)

Combine remaining 6 ingredients in small bowl. Add to sweet potato. Stir. Cook, uncovered, for about 10 minutes until tender and glazed. Makes about 3 cups (750 mL). Serves 4.

1 serving: 170 Calories; 6 g Total Fat (1.5 g Mono, 0 g Poly, 3.5 g Sat); 15 mg Cholesterol; 29 g Carbohydrate; 3 g Fibre; 2 g Protein; 210 mg Sodium

Pictured on page 53.

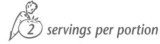 *servings per portion*

Hazelnut Acorn Squash

This easy recipe makes good use of your microwave for a quick cooking time. A sprinkle of hazelnuts and a drizzle of balsamic vinegar add plenty of character to tender squash.

Balsamic vinegar	1/4 cup	60 mL
Liquid honey	1/4 cup	60 mL
Ground allspice	1/8 tsp.	0.5 mL
Cayenne pepper, sprinkle		
Small acorn squash (about 1 lb., 454 g, each)	2	2
Water	1/4 cup	60 mL
Salt	1/4 tsp.	1 mL
Chopped flaked hazelnuts (filberts), toasted (see Tip, page 38)	3 tbsp.	45 mL

Combine first 4 ingredients in small saucepan. Bring to a boil, stirring occasionally. Reduce heat to medium. Boil gently, uncovered, for about 7 minutes until reduced by half. Remove from heat. Cool.

Cut squash in half lengthwise (see Tip, page 33). Remove and discard seeds. Cut each half into 3 wedges. Arrange in large microwave-safe dish. Add water. Microwave, covered, on high for about 10 minutes until tender (see Tip, page 119). Drain. Arrange squash, skin-side down, on large platter.

Sprinkle with salt. Drizzle with vinegar mixture.

Scatter hazelnuts over top. Makes 12 wedges. Serves 6.

1 serving: 120 Calories; 1.5 g Total Fat (1 g Mono, 0 g Poly, 0 g Sat); 0 mg Cholesterol; 29 g Carbohydrate; 4 g Fibre; 2 g Protein; 80 mg Sodium

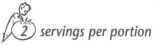

Pepper Mushroom Lentils

This earthy combination of lentils and mushrooms is brightened by the addition of lemon and red pepper. Simply stellar!

Cooking oil	2 tsp.	10 mL
Diced onion	1 cup	250 mL
Chopped portobello mushrooms	2 cups	500 mL
Diced red pepper	2 cups	500 mL
Can of lentils, rinsed and drained	19 oz.	540 mL
Grated lemon zest (see Tip, page 97)	1 tsp.	5 mL
Salt	1/2 tsp.	2 mL
Pepper	1/2 tsp.	2 mL
Grated Parmesan cheese	2 tbsp.	30 mL
Lemon juice	1 tbsp.	15 mL
Chopped fresh thyme	2 tsp.	10 mL

Heat cooking oil in large frying pan on medium. Add onion. Cook for about 5 minutes, stirring often, until softened.

Add mushrooms and red pepper. Cook for about 5 minutes, stirring occasionally, until red pepper is tender-crisp.

Add next 4 ingredients. Cook for about 2 minutes, stirring often, until heated through.

Add remaining 3 ingredients. Stir. Makes about 5 cups (1.25 L). Serves 6.

1 serving: 120 Calories; 2.5 g Total Fat (1 g Mono, 0.5 g Poly, 0.5 g Sat); trace Cholesterol; 17 g Carbohydrate; 7 g Fibre; 8 g Protein; 300 mg Sodium

 tip   Because the gills can sometimes be bitter, make sure to remove them from the portobellos. First remove the stems. Then, using a small spoon, scrape out and discard the gills.

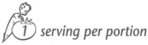

Cheesy Potato Puffs

No puffery here—just delicious cheese and herb flavour. These handy little potato puffs are fun finger food that no child will be able to resist.

Chopped peeled potato	3 cups	750 mL
Salt	1/2 tsp.	2 mL
Large egg, fork-beaten	1	1
Grated Italian cheese blend	1/3 cup	75 mL
Mayonnaise	2 tbsp.	30 mL
Italian seasoning	1/2 tsp.	2 mL
Pepper	1/8 tsp.	0.5 mL
Crushed seasoned croutons	2/3 cup	150 mL

Cooking spray

Pour water into large saucepan until about 1 inch (2.5 cm) deep. Add potato and salt. Cover. Bring to a boil. Reduce heat to medium. Boil gently for 12 to 15 minutes until tender. Drain. Mash. Let stand until cool enough to handle.

Combine next 5 ingredients in large bowl. Add potato. Stir well. Roll into 1 inch (2.5 cm) balls.

Roll balls in croutons in shallow bowl until coated. Arrange on greased baking sheet with sides. Discard any remaining croutons.

Spray with cooking spray. Bake in 350°F (175°C) oven for about 30 minutes until golden. Makes about 62 puffs. Serves 6.

1 serving: 120 Calories; 6 g Total Fat (0.5 g Mono, 0 g Poly, 1.5 g Sat); 30 mg Cholesterol; 12 g Carbohydrate; 1 g Fibre; 3 g Protein; 280 mg Sodium

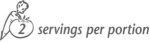

Sambal Beans

A simple green bean side with lots of heat from sambal oelek that won't overpower. Serve with your favourite Thai curry.

Cooking oil	2 tsp.	10 mL
Halved fresh (or frozen) whole green beans	6 cups	1.5 L
Finely chopped onion	1/4 cup	60 mL
Garlic cloves, minced	2	2
(or 1/2 tsp., 2 mL, powder)		
Water	1/3 cup	75 mL
Chili paste (sambal oelek)	1 tbsp.	15 mL
Soy sauce	2 tsp.	10 mL
Granulated sugar	1 tsp.	5 mL

Heat cooking oil in large frying pan on medium. Add next 3 ingredients. Heat and stir for 3 minutes.

Add water. Cook, covered, for about 7 minutes until beans are tender-crisp.

Add remaining 3 ingredients. Heat and stir for about 1 minute until glazed. Makes about 6 cups (1.5 L). Serves 6.

1 serving: 50 Calories; 1.5 g Total Fat (1 g Mono, 0 g Poly, 0 g Sat); 0 mg Cholesterol; 7 g Carbohydrate; 3 g Fibre; 2 g Protein; 170 mg Sodium

 servings per portion

Glazed Sprouts

Roasted Brussels sprouts with a simple, sweet glaze that highlights their natural flavour.

Fresh (or frozen) Brussels sprouts, larger ones halved (see Tip, page 105)	4 cups	1 L
Cooking oil	1 tbsp.	15 mL
Salt	1/4 tsp.	1 mL
Pepper	1/4 tsp.	1 mL
Apple juice	1/3 cup	75 mL
Balsamic vinegar	2 tbsp.	30 mL

(continued on next page)

Toss first 4 ingredients in large bowl until coated. Arrange in single layer on greased baking sheet with sides. Cook, uncovered, in 400°F (200°C) oven for about 20 minutes, stirring at halftime, until tender and starting to brown. Transfer to serving bowl. Cover to keep warm.

Combine apple juice and vinegar in small frying pan. Bring to a boil. Reduce heat to medium. Boil gently for about 5 minutes, stirring occasionally, until reduced and slightly thickened. Drizzle over Brussels sprouts. Toss until coated. Makes about 2 1/2 cups (625 mL). Serves 4.

1 serving: 100 Calories; 4 g Total Fat (2 g Mono, 1 g Poly, 0 g Sat); 0 mg Cholesterol; 15 g Carbohydrate; 5 g Fibre; 4 g Protein; 150 mg Sodium

 servings per portion

Ginger Bok Choy and Carrot

Simple, delicious and versatile. Bok choy pairs with carrot in a sweet ginger sauce.

Ginger marmalade	2 tbsp.	30 mL
Water	1 tbsp.	15 mL
Cornstarch	2 tsp.	10 mL
Soy sauce	2 tsp.	10 mL
Sesame oil (for flavour)	1 tsp.	5 mL
White vinegar	1/2 tsp.	2 mL
Cooking oil	1 tbsp.	15 mL
Sliced bok choy	8 cups	2 L
Thinly sliced carrot, cut diagonally	2 cups	500 mL
Roasted sesame seeds	2 tsp.	10 mL

Combine first 6 ingredients in small bowl.

Heat large frying pan or wok on medium-high until very hot. Add cooking oil. Add bok choy and carrot. Stir-fry for about 5 minutes until vegetables are tender-crisp. Stir cornstarch mixture. Add to bok choy mixture. Stir-fry for about 1 minute until boiling and thickened.

Sprinkle with sesame seeds. Stir. Makes about 4 cups (1 L). Serves 4.

1 serving: 100 Calories; 5 g Total Fat (3 g Mono, 2 g Poly, 0.5 g Sat); 0 mg Cholesterol; 12 g Carbohydrate; 3 g Fibre; 3 g Protein; 270 mg Sodium

Zucchini Parsnip Ginger Cake

Adorned with colourful bits of raisins and veggies, this spice cake has a lovely cream-cheesy glaze.

All-purpose flour	2 cups	500 mL
Brown sugar, packed	1 cup	250 mL
Minced crystallized ginger	1/4 cup	60 mL
Baking soda	1 1/2 tsp.	7 mL
Baking powder	1 tsp.	5 mL
Ground cinnamon	1 tsp.	5 mL
Ground allspice	1/2 tsp.	2 mL
Salt	1/2 tsp.	2 mL
Large eggs, fork-beaten	3	3
Grated zucchini (with peel)	1 1/2 cups	375 mL
Raisins	1 cup	250 mL
Grated parsnip	1/2 cup	125 mL
Unsweetened applesauce	1/2 cup	125 mL
Cooking oil	1/3 cup	75 mL

ORANGE CREAM CHEESE GLAZE

Block cream cheese, softened	4 oz.	125 g
Icing (confectioner's) sugar	1/2 cup	125 mL
Orange juice	2 tbsp.	30 mL
Grated orange zest (see Tip, page 97)	1/2 tsp.	2 mL

Combine first 8 ingredients in large bowl. Make a well in centre.

Combine next 6 ingredients in medium bowl. Add to well. Stir until just moistened. Spread in greased 10 cup (2.5 L) Bundt pan. Bake in 350°F (175°C) oven for about 40 minutes until wooden pick inserted in centre comes out clean. Let stand in pan for 10 minutes before removing to wire rack to cool. Place on serving plate.

Orange Cream Cheese Glaze: Beat all 4 ingredients in medium bowl until smooth. Makes about 2/3 cup (150 mL). Drizzle over top of cake, allowing glaze to flow down sides. Cuts into 16 pieces.

1 piece: 240 Calories; 8 g Total Fat (3 g Mono, 1.5 g Poly, 2 g Sat); 35 mg Cholesterol; 40 g Carbohydrate; 1 g Fibre; 3 g Protein; 240 mg Sodium

Pictured on page 143.

Avocado Coconut Squares

Avocado is good for much more than just guacamole. This layered dessert features refreshing avocado and lime with a sweet whipped cream topping.

Graham cracker crumbs	1 1/2 cups	375 mL
Butter (or hard margarine), melted	1/3 cup	75 mL
Granulated sugar	3 tbsp.	45 mL
Lime juice	1/3 cup	75 mL
Water	2 tbsp.	30 mL
Envelope of unflavoured gelatin (about 2 1/4 tsp., 11 mL)	1/4 oz.	7 g
Mashed avocado (about 4 medium)	2 cups	500 mL
Can of sweetened condensed milk	11 oz.	300 mL
Medium unsweetened coconut, toasted (see Tip, page 38)	2 tbsp.	30 mL
Grated lime zest (see Tip, page 97)	1/2 tsp.	2 mL
Whipping cream	1/2 cup	125 mL
Sour cream	1/3 cup	75 mL
Medium unsweetened coconut, toasted (see Tip, page 38)	1 tbsp.	15 mL

Combine first 3 ingredients in medium bowl. Press firmly into greased 9 x 9 inch (23 x 23 cm) pan. Bake in 375°F (190°C) oven for about 10 minutes until golden. Let stand on wire rack until cool.

Combine lime juice and water in small saucepan. Sprinkle with gelatin. Let stand for 1 minute. Heat and stir on low until gelatin is dissolved. Transfer to blender or food processor.

Add next 4 ingredients. Process, scraping down sides if necessary, until smooth. Spread evenly over crust. Chill, covered, for about 2 hours until almost set.

Beat whipping cream and sour cream in medium bowl until stiff peaks form. Spread evenly over avocado mixture. Sprinkle with second amount of coconut. Chill for about 1 hour until set. Cuts into 16 squares.

1 square: 230 Calories; 14 g Total Fat (5 g Mono, 1 g Poly, 7 g Sat); 30 mg Cholesterol; 23 g Carbohydrate; 3 g Fibre; 3 g Protein; 130 mg Sodium

Pictured on page 143.

Chocolate Surprise Pie

Yummy chocolate pudding pie—with a virtually undetectable dose of sweet potato. Delicious chocolate and orange flavours.

Can of sweet potatoes, drained	19 oz.	540 mL
Milk	1 1/4 cups	300 mL
Box of instant chocolate pudding powder	1	1
(6-serving size)		
Grated orange zest	1 tsp.	5 mL
Chocolate crumb crust	1	1
(9 inch, 23 cm, diameter)		
Whipping cream	1/2 cup	125 mL
Granulated sugar	2 tbsp.	30 mL
Vanilla extract	1/2 tsp.	2 mL
Chocolate sprinkles	1 tsp.	5 mL

Process first 4 ingredients in blender or food processor until smooth.

Pour into crust. Spread evenly. Chill, covered, for about 1 hour until set.

Beat next 3 ingredients in medium bowl until stiff peaks form. Spread over chocolate mixture.

Scatter sprinkles over top. Cuts into 8 wedges.

1 wedge: 360 Calories; 15 g Total Fat (6 g Mono, 2.5 g Poly, 6 g Sat); 20 mg Cholesterol; 55 g Carbohydrate; 2 g Fibre; 5 g Protein; 560 mg Sodium

1. Carrot Orange Custards, page 147
2. Avocado Coconut Squares, page 141
3. Zucchini Parsnip Ginger Cake, page 140

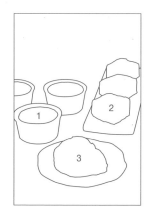

Desserts

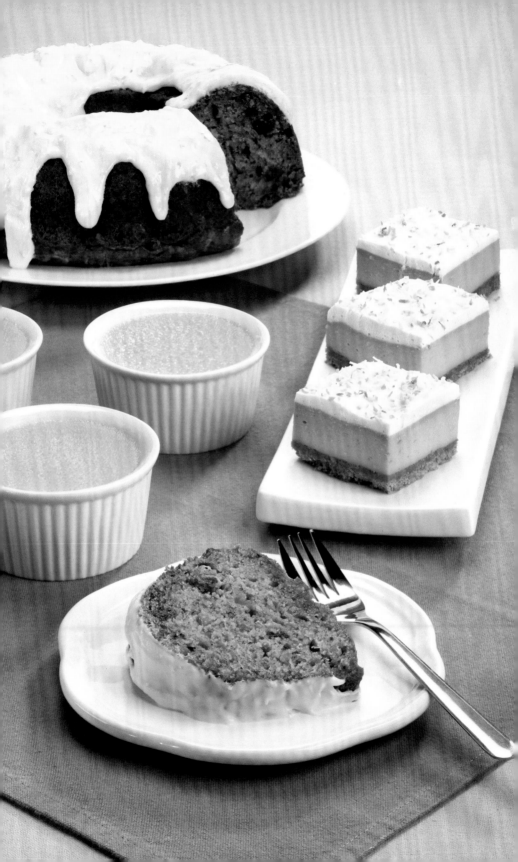

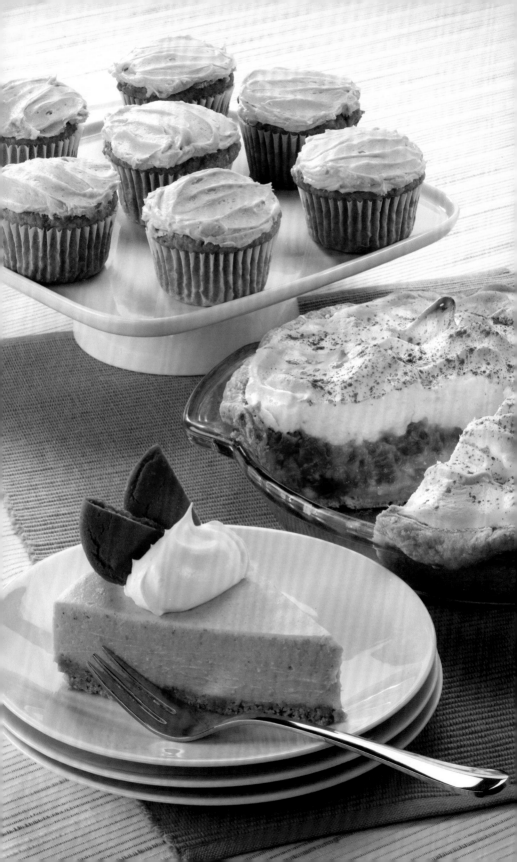

Cucumber Lemon Grass Granita

Grab a glass of this lovely slushy granita—very refreshing with cucumber,
lemon grass and a little raspberry sweetness.

Coarsely chopped, peeled and seeded English cucumber	3 1/2 cups	875 mL
Fresh (or frozen) raspberries	1 cup	250 mL
Water	1 cup	250 mL
Granulated sugar	1/2 cup	125 mL
Chopped lemon grass, bulb only	4 tsp.	20 mL

Process cucumber and raspberries in food processor until smooth.

Combine remaining 3 ingredients in small saucepan. Heat and stir on
medium until sugar is dissolved. Bring to a boil. Reduce heat to
medium-low. Simmer, covered, for 5 minutes. Add cucumber mixture. Stir.
Strain through sieve into large bowl. Discard solids. Pour into ungreased
9 x 13 inch (23 x 33 cm) pan. Freeze, covered, for 1 hour. Rake top of
mixture with fork. Repeat every hour for about 3 hours until set. Serve in
small glasses with spoons. Makes about 6 cups (1.5 L).

1/2 cup (125 mL): 40 Calories; 0 g Total Fat (0 g Mono, 0 g Poly, 0 g Sat); 0 mg Cholesterol;
10 g Carbohydrate; trace Fibre; 0 g Protein; 0 mg Sodium

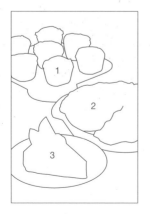

1. Spiced Eggplant Cupcakes, page 148
2. Rhubarb Meringue Pie, page 146
3. Pumpkin Mousse Cheesecake, page 151

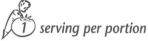

Rhubarb Meringue Pie

Delicious and creamy rhubarb custard hides beneath a golden meringue topping. Sweet and slightly tart.

Pastry for 9 inch (23 cm) deep dish pie shell

Granulated sugar	1 1/4 cups	300 mL
All-purpose flour	1/4 cup	60 mL
Egg yolks (large)	4	4
Sour cream	1/2 cup	125 mL
Vanilla extract	1 tsp.	5 mL
Chopped fresh (or frozen, thawed and drained) rhubarb	4 cups	1 L
Egg whites (large), see Safety Tip	4	4
Cream of tartar	1/4 tsp.	1 mL
Granulated sugar	1/3 cup	75 mL

Ground cinnamon, sprinkle

Roll out pastry on lightly floured surface to about 1/8 inch (3 mm) thickness. Line 9 inch (23 cm) deep dish pie plate with pastry. Trim, leaving 1/2 inch (12 mm) overhang. Roll under and crimp decorative edge.

Combine sugar and flour in large bowl. Add next 3 ingredients. Stir well.

Add rhubarb. Stir. Spread evenly in pie shell. Bake on bottom rack in 425°F (220°C) oven for 15 minutes. Reduce heat to 375°F (190°C). Bake for about 45 minutes until crust is golden.

Beat egg whites and cream of tartar in medium bowl until soft peaks form. Add sugar, 1 tbsp. (15 mL) at a time, beating constantly, until stiff peaks form and sugar is dissolved. Spread over hot pie, making sure to seal completely.

Sprinkle with cinnamon. Bake for about 10 minutes until meringue is golden. Let stand on wire rack until cool. Cuts into 8 wedges. Serves 8.

1 serving: 360 Calories; 13 g Total Fat (5 g Mono, 2.5 g Poly, 4.5 g Sat); 110 mg Cholesterol; 57 g Carbohydrate; 2 g Fibre; 6 g Protein; 160 mg Sodium

Pictured on page 144.

(continued on next page)

Safety Tip: The meringue in this recipe contains uncooked egg. Make sure to use fresh, clean Grade A eggs that are free of cracks. Keep chilled and consume the same day it is prepared. Always discard leftovers. Pregnant women, young children and the elderly are not advised to eat anything containing raw egg.

Carrot Orange Custards

Pretty orange custards with light flavour and a creamy texture.
This make-ahead dessert is perfect for company.

Chopped carrot	3/4 cup	175 mL
Ice water		
Egg yolks (large)	6	6
Granulated sugar	1/2 cup	125 mL
Vanilla extract	1/2 tsp.	2 mL
Whipping cream	2 cups	500 mL
Grated orange zest	1/2 tsp.	2 mL

Arrange six 3/4 cup (175 mL) ramekins in ungreased 9 x 13 inch (23 x 33 cm) pan. Set aside. Pour water into small saucepan until about 1 inch (2.5 cm) deep. Add carrot. Cover. Bring to a boil. Reduce heat to medium. Boil gently for about 10 minutes until tender. Drain.

Plunge carrot into ice water in medium bowl. Let stand for 5 minutes until cold. Drain. Transfer to blender or food processor.

Add next 3 ingredients. Process until smooth. Transfer to large bowl.

Heat whipping cream and zest in small saucepan on medium until hot, but not boiling. Remove from heat. Whisk 2 tbsp. (30 mL) cream mixture into egg yolk mixture. Slowly add egg yolk mixture to remaining cream mixture, whisking constantly. Pour into prepared ramekins. Pour boiling water into pan until water comes halfway up sides of ramekins. Bake in 325°F (160°C) oven for about 35 minutes until custard is set along edges but centre still wobbles. Carefully transfer ramekins to wire rack to cool completely. Chill, covered, for at least 6 hours or overnight. Makes 6 custards.

1 custard: 360 Calories; 30 g Total Fat (9 g Mono, 1.5 g Poly, 18 g Sat); 300 mg Cholesterol; 21 g Carbohydrate; 0 g Fibre; 4 g Protein; 45 mg Sodium

Pictured on page 143.

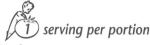
1 serving per portion

Jicama Pear Crisp

A warmly flavoured crisp with comforting spices. Jicama adds a slightly crispy texture. Perfect with ice cream or frozen yogurt.

Chopped peeled pear	3 cups	750 mL
Diced peeled jicama	3 cups	750 mL
Brown sugar, packed	1/3 cup	75 mL
Orange juice	2 tbsp.	30 mL
All-purpose flour	1 tbsp.	15 mL
Ground ginger	1/2 tsp.	2 mL
Ground cinnamon	1/4 tsp.	1 mL
Ground nutmeg	1/8 tsp.	0.5 mL
All-purpose flour	1 cup	250 mL
Quick-cooking rolled oats	1 cup	250 mL
Butter (or hard margarine), melted	3/4 cup	175 mL
Brown sugar, packed	1/2 cup	125 mL
Chopped walnuts, toasted (see Tip, page 38)	1/3 cup	75 mL
Grated orange zest (see Tip, page 97)	1/2 tsp.	2 mL
Salt	1/8 tsp.	0.5 mL

Combine first 8 ingredients in large bowl. Transfer to greased 8 x 8 inch (20 x 20 cm) baking dish.

Combine remaining 7 ingredients in medium bowl. Sprinkle over jicama mixture. Bake in 350°F (175°C) oven for about 45 minutes until topping is golden. Serves 6.

1 serving: 560 Calories; 29 g Total Fat (7 g Mono, 4.5 g Poly, 15 g Sat); 60 mg Cholesterol; 71 g Carbohydrate; 8 g Fibre; 6 g Protein; 220 mg Sodium

Spiced Eggplant Cupcakes

Having trouble getting the kids to eat their veggies? Hide five servings of vegetables in a batch of these cute cupcakes! These surprising little cakes are light, spicy and topped with a fluffy icing for the perfect finishing touch.

Chopped peeled Asian eggplant	2 1/2 cups	625 mL
Cooking oil	1 tbsp.	15 mL

(continued on next page)

Orange juice	1/2 cup	125 mL
Vanilla extract	1 tsp.	5 mL
All-purpose flour	1 1/2 cups	375 mL
Baking powder	1 tsp.	5 mL
Baking soda	1/2 tsp.	2 mL
Ground coriander	1/2 tsp.	2 mL
Ground nutmeg	1/8 tsp.	0.5 mL
Salt	1/8 tsp.	0.5 mL
Butter (or hard margarine), softened	1/3 cup	75 mL
Brown sugar, packed	3/4 cup	175 mL
Large eggs, fork-beaten	2	2
ICING		
Icing (confectioner's) sugar	1 1/4 cups	300 mL
Butter (or hard margarine), softened	1/3 cup	75 mL
Frozen concentrated grape juice, thawed	4 tsp.	20 mL

Toss eggplant and cooking oil in large bowl. Arrange in single layer on greased baking sheet with sides. Bake in 375°F (190°C) oven for about 25 minutes, stirring occasionally, until tender and starting to brown. Cool. Transfer to blender.

Add orange juice and vanilla. Process until smooth.

Combine next 6 ingredients in medium bowl.

Beat first amount of butter and brown sugar in large bowl until light and fluffy.

Add eggs, 1 at a time, beating well after each addition. Add eggplant mixture. Beat well. Add flour mixture. Stir until just combined. Fill 12 paper-lined muffin cups 3/4 full. Bake in 350°F (175°C) oven for about 18 minutes until wooden pick inserted in centre of cupcake comes out clean. Let stand in pan for 5 minutes before removing to wire racks to cool completely.

Icing: Beat all 3 ingredients on low in small bowl until smooth. Beat on high for about 3 minutes until light and fluffy. Spread over cupcakes. Makes 12 cupcakes.

1 cupcake: 280 Calories; 12 g Total Fat (3.5 g Mono, 1 g Poly, 7 g Sat); 50 mg Cholesterol; 39 g Carbohydrate; 1 g Fibre; 3 g Protein; 180 mg Sodium

Pictured on page 144.

Can't Beet Brownies

Everyone knows it doesn't get any better than brownies—and no one will ever suspect the secret addition of beet into these delightful cake-like treats.

Can of sliced beets, drained and chopped	14 oz.	398 mL
All-purpose flour	1 1/4 cups	300 mL
Granulated sugar	1 cup	250 mL
Cocoa, sifted if lumpy	1/2 cup	125 mL
Baking powder	1 tsp.	5 mL
Salt	1/4 tsp.	1 mL
Semi-sweet chocolate baking squares (1 oz., 28 g, each), chopped	2	2
Large eggs	2	2
Buttermilk (or soured milk, see Tip, page 60)	1/2 cup	125 mL
Cooking oil	1/4 cup	60 mL
Vanilla extract	1 tsp.	5 mL
Ground cinnamon	1/2 tsp.	2 mL
Ground allspice	1/8 tsp.	0.5 mL
Semi-sweet chocolate chips	1/2 cup	125 mL
Sour cream	1/4 cup	60 mL

Process beets in food processor, scraping down sides if necessary, until smooth.

Combine next 5 ingredients in medium bowl. Make a well in centre.

Microwave baking squares in small microwave-safe bowl on medium, stirring every 30 seconds, until almost melted (see Tip, page 119). Stir until smooth. Add to food processor.

Add next 6 ingredients. Process until smooth. Add to well. Stir until just moistened. Spread evenly in greased 9 x 9 inch (23 x 23 cm) pan. Bake in 350°F (175°C) oven for about 30 minutes until wooden pick inserted in centre comes out moist but not wet with batter. Do not overbake. Cool.

Place chocolate chips and sour cream in separate small microwave-safe bowl. Microwave on medium, stirring every 30 seconds, until almost melted. Stir until smooth. Spread over brownies. Let stand in pan on wire rack until cool. Cuts into 36 squares.

(continued on next page)

 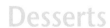

1 square: 80 Calories; 3.5 g Total Fat (1.5 g Mono, 0 g Poly, 1 g Sat); 10 mg Cholesterol; 13 g Carbohydrate; trace Fibre; 1 g Protein; 40 mg Sodium

Pumpkin Mousse Cheesecake

Rich pumpkin mousse tops a yummy gingersnap crust. This no-bake dessert is a lovely alternative to traditional pumpkin pie.

Crushed gingersnaps (about 45 gingersnaps)	2 cups	500 mL
Butter (or hard margarine), melted	1/2 cup	125 mL
Maple syrup	1/3 cup	75 mL
Water	3 tbsp.	45 mL
Envelopes of unflavoured gelatin (1/4 oz., 7 g, each)	2	2
Block cream cheese, softened	8 oz.	250 g
Can of pumpkin pie filling	19 oz.	540 mL
Ground cinnamon	1/2 tsp.	2 mL
Whipping cream	1 cup	250 mL

Halved gingersnaps, for garnish

Combine crushed gingersnaps and butter in medium bowl. Press firmly into bottom of ungreased 9 inch (23 cm) springform pan. Chill.

Combine syrup and water in small saucepan. Sprinkle with gelatin. Let stand for 1 minute. Heat and stir on low until gelatin is dissolved.

Beat cream cheese in large bowl until smooth. Add pumpkin pie filling and cinnamon. Beat well. Slowly add gelatin mixture, beating constantly until smooth.

Beat whipping cream in small bowl until stiff peaks form. Fold half into pumpkin mixture. Chill remaining whipped cream. Spread pumpkin mixture evenly over crust. Chill, covered, for about 3 hours until set.

Garnish with halved gingersnaps and remaining whipped cream. Cuts into 12 wedges.

1 wedge: 340 Calories; 23 g Total Fat (4.5 g Mono, 1 g Poly, 13 g Sat); 65 mg Cholesterol; 34 g Carbohydrate; 4 g Fibre; 4 g Protein; 350 mg Sodium

Pictured on page 144.

Measurement Tables

Throughout this book measurements are given in Conventional and Metric measure. To compensate for differences between the two measurements due to rounding, a full metric measure is not always used. The cup used is the standard 8 fluid ounce. Temperature is given in degrees Fahrenheit and Celsius. Baking pan measurements are in inches and centimetres as well as quarts and litres. An exact metric conversion is given below as well as the working equivalent (Metric Standard Measure).

Spoons

Conventional Measure	Metric Exact Conversion Millilitre (mL)	Metric Standard Measure Millilitre (mL)
1/8 teaspoon (tsp.)	0.6 mL	0.5 mL
1/4 teaspoon (tsp.)	1.2 mL	1 mL
1/2 teaspoon (tsp.)	2.4 mL	2 mL
1 teaspoon (tsp.)	4.7 mL	5 mL
2 teaspoons (tsp.)	9.4 mL	10 mL
1 tablespoon (tbsp.)	14.2 mL	15 mL

Cups

Conventional Measure	Metric Exact Conversion Millilitre (mL)	Metric Standard Measure Millilitre (mL)
1/4 cup (4 tbsp.)	56.8 mL	60 mL
1/3 cup (5 1/3 tbsp.)	75.6 mL	75 mL
1/2 cup (8 tbsp.)	113.7 mL	125 mL
2/3 cup (10 2/3 tbsp.)	151.2 mL	150 mL
3/4 cup (12 tbsp.)	170.5 mL	175 mL
1 cup (16 tbsp.)	227.3 mL	250 mL
4 1/2 cups	1022.9 mL	1000 mL (1 L)

Oven Temperatures

Fahrenheit (°F)	Celsius (°C)
175°	80°
200°	95°
225°	110°
250°	120°
275°	140°
300°	150°
325°	160°
350°	175°
375°	190°
400°	200°
425°	220°
450°	230°
475°	240°
500°	260°

Dry Measurements

Conventional Measure Ounces (oz.)	Metric Exact Conversion Grams (g)	Metric Standard Measure Grams (g)
1 oz.	28.3 g	28 g
2 oz.	56.7 g	57 g
3 oz.	85.0 g	85 g
4 oz.	113.4 g	125 g
5 oz.	141.7 g	140 g
6 oz.	170.1 g	170 g
7 oz.	198.4 g	200 g
8 oz.	226.8 g	250 g
16 oz.	453.6 g	500 g
32 oz.	907.2 g	1000 g (1 kg)

Pans

Conventional Inches	Metric Centimetres
8x8 inch	20x20 cm
9x9 inch	23x23 cm
9x13 inch	23x33 cm
10x15 inch	25x38 cm
11x17 inch	28x43 cm
8x2 inch round	20x5 cm
9x2 inch round	23x5 cm
10x4 1/2 inch tube	25x11 cm
8x4x3 inch loaf	20x10x7.5 cm
9x5x3 inch loaf	23x12.5x7.5 cm

Casseroles

CANADA & BRITAIN		UNITED STATES	
Standard Size Casserole	Exact Metric Measure	Standard Size Casserole	Exact Metric Measure
1 qt. (5 cups)	1.13 L	1 qt. (4 cups)	900 mL
1 1/2 qts. (7 1/2 cups)	1.69 L	1 1/2 qts. (6 cups)	1.35 L
2 qts. (10 cups)	2.25 L	2 qts. (8 cups)	1.8 L
2 1/2 qts. (12 1/2 cups)	2.81 L	2 1/2 qts. (10 cups)	2.25 L
3 qts. (15 cups)	3.38 L	3 qts. (12 cups)	2.7 L
4 qts. (20 cups)	4.5 L	4 qts. (16 cups)	3.6 L
5 qts. (25 cups)	5.63 L	5 qts. (20 cups)	4.5 L

Recipe Index

153

154

155

S

159

HEALTHY COOKING SERIES

To your health—and bon appétit!

You've asked and Company's Coming has listened! The new Healthy Cooking Series delivers delicious healthy recipes and nutrition information from leading health and wellness experts. These beautiful, full-colour cookbooks will transform the way you eat—and the way you live!

Now Available!

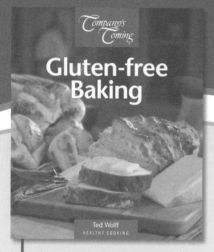

Now Available!

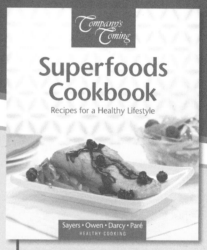

Finally—a book that shows you how to make delicious baked goods and sweets that are completely gluten-free. Ted Wolff, founder of Kinnikinnick Foods, makes living gluten-free easy in this highly requested title.

Blueberries lower your risk for cardiovascular disease, and walnuts reduce your risk of diabetes and cancer. With these recipes, you can easily add superfoods to your daily diet and improve your health and well-being.

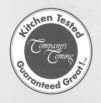

Visit our website for sample recipes and more information:

www.companyscoming.com